HEALTHY
WEIGHT
LOSS

Dr. Miriam Stoppard

HEALTHY WEIGHT LOSS

HEALTHCARE

DK PUBLISHING, INC.

Visit us on the World Wide Web at www.dk.com

A DK PUBLISHING BOOK
Visit us on the World Wide Web at www.dk.com

DESIGN AND EDITORIAL BY   Edward Kinsey and
Jacqueline Jackson

SENIOR MANAGING ART EDITOR   Lynne Brown
MANAGING EDITOR   Corinne Roberts

SENIOR ART EDITOR   Karen Ward
SENIOR EDITOR   Penny Warren
US EDITOR   Jill Hamilton

PRODUCTION   Sarah Coltman

First American Edition, 1999
2 4 6 8 10 9 7 5 3 1
Published in the United States by DK Publishing Inc.
95 Madison Avenue, New York, New York 10016
Material in this publication was previously published in
Lose 7lb in 7 Days by Dr. Miriam Stoppard
Published in Great Britain by Dorling Kindersley Limited

Stoppard, Miriam.
Healthy weight loss / by Miriam Stoppard.
p. cm. -- (DK healthcare series)
Includes index.
ISBN 0-7894-3757-0 (pbk.)
1. Weight loss. 2. Reducing diets. I. Title. II. Series.
RM222.2.S848 1998
613.2'5--dc21   98-25876
CIP

Reproduced by Colourscan, Singapore
Printed in Hong Kong by Wing King Tong

CONTENTS

INTRODUCTION 6

INTRODUCTION

I have a vested interest in a healthy eating plan because I confess that I have been overweight and a failed dieter all my life. At the age of fifty-three I finally seemed to have cracked it. For the first time I felt free from the need to diet. And I want to share my secret with you.

If you are overweight, you are unhealthy. So one of your goals is to become not only a trimmer you but a healthier you. I am not promising that you will live longer, but you are fairly sure to enjoy your life more if you are fit and trim. As a doctor, I believe that any eating plan must emphasize the long term, because with the acquisition of new eating habits, it's much easier to keep the weight off. So we have to start paying attention to what we eat, how often we eat and the ritual of eating; we have to acquire a new personal psychology of eating – not an easy job when so many bad habits have to be unlearned.

Preparation is a key factor because it will help ensure your success. Step-by-step guidelines on how to optimize your chances of success by choosing your start time carefully, by signing a contract, and by planning and shopping for the whole week will ease you into the eating plan.

If you stick to this eating plan, you could lose about 4½–6½lb (2–3kg) in seven days. Bear in mind that if you cheat on the odd occasion, it is not the end of the world. Please do not throw in the sponge as you may have done in the past. We now know that, as far as eating is concerned, the body does not work on a 24-hour clock but on a much longer timescale, probably nearer a week. This gives you lots of opportunity to make up for any minor misdemeanors.

Come on, you can do it. The key is to change the way you think. This time you will be successful – losing weight has rarely been made easier. More importantly, it has rarely made as much sense.

PREPARING TO DIET

You may be tempted to skip this chapter and go straight to the seven-day diet, but the more carefully you prepare beforehand, the more likely you are to lose weight and keep it off permanently. In this chapter, I explain how to assess your target weight, and how to keep a food diary so that you have a realistic idea of how much you eat. Motivation is crucial to healthy weight loss, so to fortify your resolve before you start my diet, I strongly suggest that you enlist the support of your family and friends and that you sign the Seven-day Contract. Good luck!

YOU AND YOUR DIET

There have long been a great many conflicting ideas about the best way to lose weight and keep it off. Here are a few facts that should help clarify the situation.

YOUR ENERGY NEEDS

If you eat more than you need, you will put on weight. The energy you require to run all the everyday processes that go on in your body is determined by the rate at which your body metabolizes at rest. This is called the basal metabolic rate (BMR). It is difficult for experts to measure your metabolic rate precisely because it is a complex business. They have to know how much oxygen you inhale and how much carbon dioxide you exhale as energy is burned in your body.

Plenty of energy is used, even at rest, because your heart beats, your diaphragm contracts and relaxes, your digestive system breaks down food and pushes it along, and thousands of other macro and micro events take place. A large amount of energy is also used to provide heat.

The average figures for the basal metabolic rate of a man or woman depend on his or her height, weight, and body composition. Body composition is especially significant and also widely misunderstood; put simply, it means lean muscle versus fat. A lean man who weighs, say, 143lb (65kg) might require about 1,500 calories a day just for his basal metabolism (in other words before doing any kind of activity). Of that, the muscles, brain, liver, kidneys, and heart will account for over four-fifths of the energy used. Since fat is not an organ, it requires very little energy to be maintained. But a fat man who weighs 143lb (65kg) would have a smaller body mass of active organs (mostly muscle), and extra fat. With less muscle and more fat, he might require only some 1,250 calories a day for his basal metabolism.

MUSCLE HELPS WEIGHT LOSS

When you are overweight, the problem is not as simple as you might think. Not only are you over your ideal weight but in addition you probably have a disproportionate amount of fat instead of muscle. The point is this: when you diet, the more muscle you lose as a percentage of your body weight, the less energy you need and this leads to a further imbalance between fat and muscle. However, if you combine a sensible diet with exercise, you will not only build up your muscle mass and tone up muscles that are out of condition, you will also raise your metabolic rate and thereby burn up more energy regardless of what you are doing. Furthermore, by exercising, whether it's brisk walking, dancing, or marathon running, you will burn up energy over and above your basal metabolic requirements, which means that, once your weight is satisfactory, you can consume more calories and still stay at your ideal weight. Exercise is therefore the key to weight loss. None of this is new information but it's surprising how easily it can be forgotten when reading the hype on some of the more unlikely diet regimens.

STOP DRASTIC DIETING, START EATING

As you can now appreciate, the amount of energy you burn daily, apart from any specific activities you undertake, is variable and you can make a positive impact on it. You can also do the opposite.

The popularity in the last few years of microdiets (diets where you consume only some 350 calories a day) has prompted concern that you will end up losing lean muscle mass rather than fat. But the most striking argument against them is their effect on the basal metabolism. If you put your body on a starvation diet, it thinks it really is starving and takes appropriate action. This action is akin to hibernation, although not quite as drastic. The body simply slows down and burns less energy. That is why a small woman who is heavily overweight can consume less than 1,000 calories a day and still put on weight, whereas another small but active woman of the same weight who eats more calories a day may actually lose weight.

My diet avoids the trap caused by extreme diets. You must eat a sensible amount each day of different kinds of foods – that is, very little fat, salt, sugar, red meat, and processed foods, but moderate amounts of poultry, eggs, and fish, and large amounts of fresh fruit and vegetables, beans, legumes, wholegrain rice, and oats. You are encouraged to exercise regularly and, what's more, by eating your food in six smaller installments you will burn off more calories than if you ate the same food as three larger meals.

SETTING A TARGET WEIGHT

In the charts (below and opposite), there is an "acceptable" weight range for each height that covers the normal variation in body shape. If you are small-framed, your ideal weight should be nearer the lower range, and if you are large-framed, your weight may be nearer the upper end of the acceptable range.

If, after consulting the charts, you find that you are overweight (and you probably knew that already), I want you to set yourself a realistic target weight as your first step toward becoming slimmer and fitter.

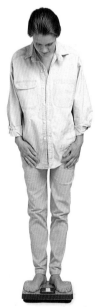

Monitor your weight
Weekly weighing will tell you whether you are actually losing weight.

GETTING STARTED

Even if you have been a failed dieter all your life, this time you are going to succeed. I've made it as easy as possible for you to follow my eating plan by supplying a shopping list, menus, and recipes for all seven days. Each day I tell you a little more about how to use healthy foods to your advantage. I also suggest muscle-toning and relaxation exercises to get you into better shape and, because you deserve it, each day there will be a treat. Finally, I have lots of tips on how to overcome cravings and stop bingeing, and on what to do if you don't think you can complete the week, or if you get the urge to cheat.

BEFORE YOU BEGIN

The first thing to do is take a good look at yourself when you're undressed. If there are bulges in the wrong places, tell yourself that soon they'll be a memory because once you've regained control of your weight you won't let yourself slip back into that situation.

Next, weigh yourself on the scales. I don't believe in overzealous weight-watching once I've started dieting because some days I lose weight and other days I don't, which can be demoralizing. The truth is, your body weight fluctuates anyway, so it's more realistic to record your weight at the beginning and the end of the week rather than day by day. Even better, find a pair of

WEIGHT RANGE CHART FOR MEN

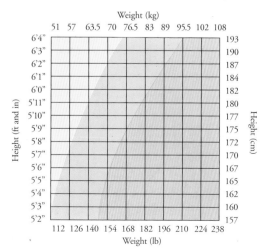

flattering jeans or some other favorite piece of clothing that's a bit too tight. Hang it up in a prominent place so that each time you weaken, you can see it hanging there waiting for you to wear again.

You should know your height, but if you don't, measure that as well. Now check yourself against the appropriate height/weight charts (below and opposite). You are overweight when you are above the acceptable weight range, and obese if you weigh 20 percent above the upper end of the acceptable range. Now set yourself a target weight to aim for (see column, opposite).

Incidentally, as a species, we don't vary in basic frame as much as some of us would like to think. In healthy people, there is no such thing as having "heavy bones" since the only people who have light bones are probably suffering from osteoporosis, literally porous bones. This is a condition that occurs in later life for some women, and can often be avoided if your normal diet contains enough calcium. This is especially important for women over the age of 35. You should also make sure you do a reasonable amount of weight-bearing exercise such as walking, running, riding, biking – even simply standing helps.

Remember, after completing my seven-day plan, if you continue to exercise and follow my advice for healthy eating, you will continue to shape up. Or you can return to the diet for a second assault on the flab at any time if you need to.

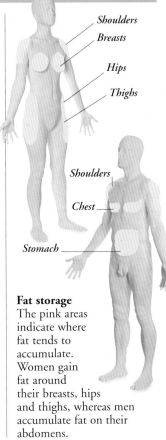

Fat storage
The pink areas indicate where fat tends to accumulate. Women gain fat around their breasts, hips and thighs, whereas men accumulate fat on their abdomens.

WEIGHT RANGE CHART FOR WOMEN

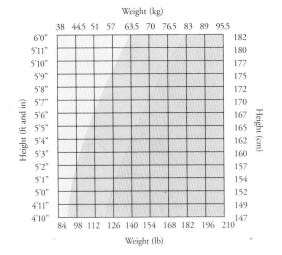

Weight (kg)

Find your weight
The charts (left and opposite) show whether your present weight is appropriate for your height and sex. First locate your height and weight along the sides of the chart, then note where they cross.

Underweight
Acceptable weight
Overweight

FAST AND FATTENING FOODS

All too often, convenience foods and calorie-rich snacks are an easily forgotten part of our daily diet.

Today, the slightest hint of a food craving is very quickly and easily appeased by wolfing down a snack. Mostly, these snacks are made with a shelf-life that suits supermarkets and the like, so that they can be kept for long periods without refrigeration or any other special storage arrangements. Unfortunately, that usually means that they have been processed and refined so much that they have lost all or most of their nutrients, leaving only sugar or salt, and calories. What's worse is that, stripped of fiber and any bulk, the sugary snacks don't sate your hunger for long! In fact, as you have no doubt noticed, they tend to make you want more.

Salty, savory snacks such as nuts, crackers, or other bar foods make your body dehydrated and make you more thirsty. Alcohol is high in calories and low in nutrients and won't help make you feel better.

That's why no convenience foods, snacks, or processed or refined food products are allowed in my seven-day eating plan.

GETTING ORGANIZED

You need to be well prepared before you start the eating plan. In order to make it as easy and painless as possible, you must first of all do some research – nothing complicated, just a careful look at exactly what your eating habits are really like.

A FOOD DIARY

Before you start the plan, keep a diary of every single thing that passes your lips for one week. Don't be tempted to cheat or overlook anything. Look out, especially, for all those nibbles in the late afternoon and early evening. Research has shown that this is often the worst time of the day for unnecessary eating. Many overweight people eat normal-sized meals at lunch and dinner time but also eat as many calories as a good-sized meal in the form of snacks around this time.

I don't like constantly counting calories – it just makes eating less of a pleasure and more of a chore – but it is worth taking a hard look at the calories you consume over a week. There are plenty of books available that will tell you the caloric value of most foods; you may even have one already if, like me, you've tried lots of diets before now.

It is quite likely that you will find that most of your high-calorie intake is in the form of snacks or alcohol. All of us can enjoy the occasional cookie, chocolate bar, or social drink, but very few of us can afford to take a large portion of our energy requirements in that form on a regular basis. If you do, your body will not be getting enough of the important nutrients it needs such as protein, minerals, and vitamins. The result is either you will eat more in order to maintain an adequate level of nutrition, or you will start to lose valuable nutrients from your body, which in practice will mean losing muscle and gaining fat. So start cutting out snacks and alcoholic drinks right now.

WHEN TO BEGIN

Once you have analyzed your food diary and identified your problem areas, you should have a better understanding of your present eating habits. You can use that information to pick the best day of the week to start my seven-day eating plan.

TIPS

- If you find you eat more food on weekends, perhaps socially as a family, don't start your diet on a weekend.
- If it's the snacks that you eat to keep you going at the office that bother you most, start on the weekend when you're free from this particular temptation.
- A useful tip for women is not to start in your premenstrual week. That's often a time when our will-power is at its lowest ebb and there's a strong desire to binge. It's also a time when a lot of women retain fluid, sometimes as much as 6lb (3kg), so it's not a good idea to be measuring weight loss.
- A good strategy must take account of the psychology behind eating. Much of the excess food we eat is not in response to hunger but simply as a form of comfort. Find other ways to make yourself feel comfortable and occupy your mind.
- One thing that helps a great many people stick to their decision to lose weight is a contract. So, if you haven't already, turn to the contract (p. 15), fill in the dates, find someone to witness it, and sign it yourself.
- If your principles will allow it, make a bet with a friend that you'll lose the weight.
- Remember to keep that favorite item of clothing in a prominent place to act as an inspiration when you're at your lowest ebb.
- Even if your partner, friends, or colleagues don't join you on the seven-day plan, be sure to tell them that you are doing it. Ask them not to tempt you with food or expect you to join them in any binges.
- When you're watching your food consumption, there's no doubt that the evenings are the hardest part of the day, so be well prepared for this. Warn friends and family alike that you will be unable to join them for dinners or at restaurants during this week.
- Even after doing your exercises and having your treat of the day, you will probably have some time on your hands, so take advantage of it and plan in advance what you will do. Go to see a movie you've been meaning to catch for ages or simply settle down to watch a favorite TV program you keep missing. Or why don't you read that book you've heard so much about?

HOW PARTNERS AND FRIENDS CAN HELP

One of the best ways to ease your way through the seven days is to follow the eating plan with someone else, or better still, try it with a group of friends. That way, you can still eat socially without having to eat separate food.

If your partner also needs to lose weight, why don't you go on the plan together? You will be able to back up each other and help out in moments of weakness.

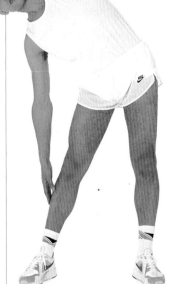

Exercising works
Dieting alone will not help you lose weight easily; you must also increase the amount of exercise you do.

REASONS TO SUCCEED

When you go on my seven-day plan, not only will you lose weight, but you will feel better and, most importantly, you will be in control.

- *For me, being fat equals being miserable, and one of the reasons we're all so miserable when we're overweight is that we feel out of control. Once you get your eating under control, you'll feel much, much happier, not only about food but about yourself. This is because:*

- *You'll stop being obsessed about food.*

- *Your self-image will improve.*

- *You'll gain confidence.*

- *The knowledge that you'll never be fat again will give you a new lease on life.*

So, believe me, it's worth it. Make the effort for yourself and no one else. You're important – give yourself the highest priority.

DIETING AND THE FAMILY

If you have to cook for your family, it shouldn't be difficult to overlap their food needs with yours. Everything on the seven-day plan is highly nutritious, and it will do them a world of good to eat plenty of fresh fruit and vegetables. If you have children who "don't like vegetables" don't despair, but also don't expect them to become converts to healthy eating overnight. Both the seven-day eating plan (see p. 25) and my guidelines for staying slim and healthy for the rest of your life (see p. 65) feature lots of food in its natural state. That means you will have much more fiber in your diet and a lot more bulk. Children need to be allowed time to adjust to this, and I suggest you introduce it little by little. I promise you it will be worth it, especially if your children eat a lot of processed or junk food at present.

Eating junk food tends to lead to extremes of mood because it makes blood sugar levels rise then drop dramatically. As your children are converted to eating less processed food, you may notice their moods don't fluctuate quite so dramatically. This is because they're getting a much steadier supply of energy – a natural slow-release system – and also a more reliable supply of all the nutrients they need.

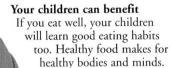

Your children can benefit
If you eat well, your children will learn good eating habits too. Healthy food makes for healthy bodies and minds.

MY SEVEN-DAY CONTRACT

I have decided to start on a new eating plan.

I will decide when I am going to start and mark it in my diary.

I will make my decision public and tell my family, friends, and colleagues.
I will try to get their support.

I will follow the seven-day eating plan precisely, without cheating, and I will lose approximately 6lb (3kg) in weight.

I shall seek help from ....

.... [insert name of partner or friend]
who will encourage me at all times to stick to the eating plan, and whom I can call on for support.

I shall weigh myself on ....
and not weigh myself again until the seven days are over.

.... [date]

At the end of seven days I will get into my favorite jeans/dress/swimsuit.

I will undertake all of these actions:

Signed ....

Witnessed ....

Signed ....

Witnessed .... [Sponsor]
....

RELAXATION AND EXERCISE

Every evening of the seven-day plan, I want you to do these simple relaxation exercises. They will help you get in tune with your body and by doing so become more relaxed. Don't attempt too much at first, but as the exercises become easier, do more of them until you have a daily routine that incorporates them all.

To start, try deep breathing. First take a deep breath in through your nose to the count of four. When you think you've drawn all the air you can into your lungs, take in another little sharp breath, and then relax and breathe out through your mouth. Keep exhaling until you feel empty, then a little more to squeeze that last breath out. Feel yourself relaxing each time you breathe out. Feel that oxygen filling up your lungs and feel it flowing around your body. Do this at least five times. You can do it when you are ready for bed or anywhere else; try it whenever you just want to feel more relaxed.

Next, build on this breathing routine with some deep muscle relaxation. Find a quiet place that's comfortable, such as the bedroom. Lie down and close your eyes. Concentrate on your right hand if you are right-handed, or your left if you are left-handed. Make as tight a fist as you can, and then relax it. This makes you aware of how relaxed you want to be. Now concentrate on making your hand feel warm and heavy. Repeat it to yourself: "warm and heavy." Let your whole arm become warm and heavy. Then let the arm go and feel it sink into the bed or floor. Now repeat the exercise for your other hand and arm. Concentrate on each foot and leg in turn, feeling your lower leg and then your thigh become warm and heavy. Carry the sensation up into your buttocks and abdomen, letting them all sink into the bed or floor. Now do your chest and finally your jaw, neck, and mouth. Finish by telling yourself to be cool, cool.

If you haven't done relaxation techniques before, don't expect to master them in one attempt and don't rush them. Practice this routine for 15 or 20 minutes every day if you can; even a few minutes, if that's all the time you can take, is better than nothing.

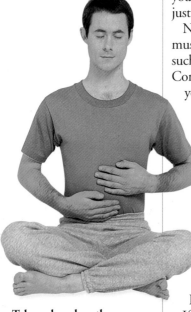

Take a deep breath
Breathing deeply and slowly while emptying your mind can help you relax and regain your poise. Be sure to sit or lie in a comfortable position.

After you have mastered the deep muscle relaxation exercises, try some mental relaxation and positive imagery. This will help you combat stressful thoughts and concerns and will enable you to take control of your body. As before, start with some deep breathing, then I want you to do some free association.

Let your mind flit from one thought to another. Think of something positive and pleasant and just follow a line of thought wherever it takes you. If an unpleasant thought comes into your head, say "no" and keep it out. The color blue is a relaxing color. You could think of a blue sky and a blue sea. Or picture a field of waving corn. Think about your breathing, feel the air filling your lungs, and then breathe out slowly and relax.

Remember to find a quiet and comfortable place without distractions and start with the deep breathing. Make time each day for these relaxation techniques and you will find that you become less bothered by stress and worrying.

HOW EXERCISE HELPS

Many people dislike the thought of having to exercise as part of a weight-loss program. But in my seven-day plan I have made it easy for you to incorporate exercise gradually into your daily routine. Over one week, I encourage you to be more physically active, and show you how to tone specific parts of your body by doing simple exercises. I've suggested a realistic number of repetitions for each type of exercise; once you achieve these targets, you can set yourself new goals. Since most people have a busy life, I have made sure that no single activity is too time-consuming. Each activity will either form part of your daily routine anyway, for example, walking up the stairs instead of taking the elevator, or it will be a simple exercise you can do while you watch television or listen to music. And if you find that you are making excuses not to do your daily exercise, remember that the sooner you've done it, the sooner you can begin your daily treat!

Continuing to exercise Once you have completed the seven-day plan, you can use the simple exercises I have suggested as a basis for creating a program that is right for you. For example, you may decide to spend one day

Bike to fitness
Biking is an excellent aerobic exercise: it raises your heart rate as well as strengthening your leg muscles.

17

EXERCISE TIPS

To make exercising as easy and safe as possible, follow these general tips:

• *If you are very unfit or overweight, before beginning any sort of exercise program, check with your doctor that it is safe to do so.*

• *If you join a health club, make sure that you are given thorough instructions on how to use the equipment.*

• *Always do some simple stretching before exercising to warm up, and afterward to cool down.*

• *Drink plenty of water before, during, and after exercising, especially when doing any aerobic activity.*

• *To get the most out of an aerobic activity, such as swimming, running, and biking, aim to exercise at a moderate pace for at least 20 minutes. You should be slightly breathless, but not gasping for breath.*

• *If you are feeling very fatigued or unwell, don't force yourself to exercise. Listen to your body.*

• *If at any point while exercising you feel faint or exhausted, stop immediately.*

• *Leave at least an hour between eating a heavy meal and starting your exercises.*

simply concentrating on doing the leg exercises I have outlined, and another day concentrating on toning your stomach muscles. You may decide to make aerobic exercise, such as going swimming or doing an exercise class, a weekly event. If you go with your partner or a friend, this can become an enjoyable social activity; if you go alone, it may become a time for you to get away from it all. It can be nerve-wracking going to an exercise class or gym by yourself, especially if you haven't exercised for a long time, but you'll soon get to know people. In fact, the more often you go, the easier it will become. And don't worry about what you wear – a baggy t-shirt and sweatpants are fine.

You don't have to do specific exercises every day, and you certainly shouldn't feel guilty if you miss doing a part of your regular exercise program in one particular week. I just want to encourage you to become more physically active so that, eventually, walking instead of driving, or climbing the stairs instead of taking the elevator, are activities that you do as a matter of course.

THE BENEFITS OF EXERCISE

Becoming fitter is very beneficial to your physical and emotional health. Whatever your age or level of fitness, I can guarantee that exercising regularly and being more physically active will make you feel good. This is because during exercise the body releases hormones called endorphins, which are natural antidepressants. You'll also feel great because you'll lose weight or maintain weight loss, sleep better, have more energy, be better able to cope with stress, and have improved posture.

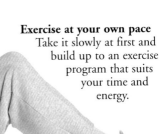

Exercise at your own pace
Take it slowly at first and build up to an exercise program that suits your time and energy.

FIVE BASIC FOODS

There are several dishes that you will be eating quite regularly when you follow the seven-day plan because they are the dieter's best friends. They are satisfying, and they depress the appetite and suppress cravings. Some of them are best made in advance, and some may not be familiar to you. Here are the basic recipes and a few serving suggestions.

Oatmeal This is my favorite breakfast. It sets you up for the rest of the day, it's nutritious, and it does you a world of good. Oats, and especially oat bran, are one of the richest sources of soluble fiber. Research has shown that regular daily helpings of oats in one form or another can actually reduce the level of cholesterol and other low density lipoproteins in our blood – over and above the effect of any special low-fat diet. Furthermore, the sticky spongelike mass of soluble fiber slows down the rate of absorption of sugar and helps keep the blood glucose levels from shooting up and down. A steadier level of blood glucose will make you feel better and you will be less likely to get cravings.

As a general rule, I don't think you should add salt to food, especially if you have high blood pressure or a heart condition, but I like a little with my oatmeal. If you aren't bothered, then don't add any! Many people have more difficulty eating oatmeal without spoonfuls of sugar or syrup. I'm afraid that is absolutely out of the question. If you like it sweet, you could use a low-calorie sweetener but, better still, use an unprocessed sweetener – fruit. It could be chopped dried fruit – apricots, raisins, and prunes are delicious. Alternatively, slice in a fresh peach or nectarine. Either way your oatmeal tastes sweeter without resorting to processed and refined ingredients.

Wholegrain rice This is one of the foods I recommend for the early evening snack meal. It's a good, nutritious source of energy in the right form – unprocessed carbohydrate. Make sure you buy wholegrain rice – it's mostly sold as brown rice. White rice has had the husk removed and has then been polished, losing most of its nutrition and fiber content.

OATMEAL FOR ONE PERSON

Ingredients
2 cups (50g) oatmeal
1¼ cups (300ml) water or skim milk
pinch of salt
skim milk to taste

Method
1 Put the oatmeal into a saucepan.
2 Add about 1¼ cups (300ml) of water or skim milk. Add a good pinch of salt to taste if you like it.
3 Bring it to a boil so that it begins to bubble, then simmer for 3 minutes, stirring all the time. Serve with up to ½ cup (50ml) skim milk.

HOW TO COOK BROWN RICE

1 It helps to begin by dry frying or cracking it in a pan. You don't need any oil: just heat the pan, add the rice, and stir. After a minute or so, the rice will crack and jump; stir vigorously so that it won't burn.

2 Once most of it is cracked, pour in the water. Recipes vary widely in the amount of water they recommend. You could use a lot, and drain the rice when it's ready.

3 Some people prefer to cook rice with only 1¼ times as much water as rice. Add boiling water and stir. Once the water has returned to a boil, stop stirring and leave it alone. Put a lid on the dish and place it in the oven for about 45 minutes at 375°F/190°C until the water is absorbed and the rice is done.

HOW TO COOK DAHL

Ingredients
1 cup (225g) lentils/split peas
1⅓ cups (300ml) water
1 small onion, finely sliced
1 clove garlic, crushed
a pinch of cumin
black pepper

Method
1 Start by soaking the lentils overnight.
2 The next day, rinse them thoroughly, add the water, and boil for 10 minutes.
3 Reduce the heat, add the finely sliced onion and garlic, and simmer until the lentils are cooked and the water absorbed. Depending on how fresh the lentils or split peas are, this could be 30 minutes or as much as 45 minutes.

If you can't wait to soak the lentils overnight, here's a quick way to make dahl:

1 Pour 5 cups (1¼ liters) of boiling water over the lentils and let them stand for one hour.
2 Drain and rinse them thoroughly.
3 Cook the lentils at high pressure in a pressure cooker for 15 minutes.
4 Reduce the pressure and continue simmering them on a stove, adding the seasoning and stirring frequently.

Be adventurous and add a variety of spices and seasonings to the rice:

• Add half a finely chopped onion to the water with a teaspoonful of black pepper and ground cumin.

• Two squashed cardamoms and a little ground turmeric will give it an authentic Indian flavor and color.

• If you like a nutty flavor, spoil yourself by adding 2 tbsp (25g) wild rice to 1¼ cups (225g) wholegrain rice. The black seeds are really grass seeds, and not rice at all, but they make the dish look and taste rather exotic.

• Another way to make rice special is to buy a little real saffron, the tiny red stamens picked from the hearts of crocuses. Add a good pinch to the rice while it's cooking, and a little more just before serving to give it a wonderful color and aroma.

Once it's cooked and cooled, keep the rice in an airtight container in the refrigerator, ready for your six o'clock dinners, but do not keep it for longer than a week.

Dahl Dahl is another excellent food that I recommend for your six o'clock snack meal. Again, once it is prepared, it can be kept in the refrigerator and you can eat a little with rice or on its own. If you've never eaten it, you have a treat in store. It's made from lentils or split peas and it's very nutritious. Like all the legumes, it is rich in protein and fiber but low in fat – just what we want.

• Don't add any salt during cooking. This is not just to cut down on salt, but also because cooking lentils in salt water makes them tougher.

• Season with generous amounts of cumin and black pepper. As a variation, try turmeric and cloves, or make a hot version with some fresh chilis. Don't be afraid to add a lot of spice – lentils need strong flavoring for best results.

• Once the lentils are cooked, stir well and you should have a delicious paste with the consistency of pease pudding (which is another food I highly recommend).

Stock Homemade stock is the secret of making delicious soups, sauces and many other meals. It's very simple to prepare (see column, opposite) and you can make it using a poultry carcass or just vegetables. If you have salad vegetables that are slightly past their prime (but not bruised or bad), this is an excellent use for them. Also, any foliage from fennel, celery, or young carrots

adds to the flavor. Be sure to include the stalks from parsley and other herbs; they contain most of the flavor.
• After you have cooled the stock in the refrigerator overnight, all the fat will have solidified as a white layer on top, which can be easily removed. What's left underneath is a wonderfully tasty and nutritious stock jelly suitable for making soups, gravies, or adding to any savory dish that uses liquid.
• A good way to store stock is to freeze it. If you are going to do this, pour it into suitable freezer containers before it has cooled and remove the fat later.
• If you don't want to use bones in your stock, you can still make a delicious sweet stock with vegetables and herbs. However, don't bother to reduce it because it will not form a jelly and prolonged boiling will remove some of the nutrients. Instead, start with less water – about 5 cups (1 liter) – depending on the size of the pot and the amount of vegetables. Incidentally, chefs call this a *court bouillon* and it is excellent for poaching vegetables and fish.
• If you have a pressure cooker, you can make stock in about 40 minutes, or 20 minutes if you're not using bones. If you don't have one, it will take a good two hours of simmering to get the best flavor.

Vegetables for soup
Homemade vegetable soups can be made from many kinds of vegetables and are a wonderful source of vitamins and fiber. Make a large batch ahead of time and store it in your refrigerator for the week.

HOW TO MAKE STOCK

Ingredients
a selection of fresh vegetables (carrots, potatoes, onions, leeks, and celery as desired)
8 cups (2 liters) water
1–2 bay leaves, sprig of fresh thyme, 12 peppercorns, rosemary, parsley
poultry bones (optional)

Method
1 Clean the vegetables and trim off any bruised parts.
2 Put your stock bones in a large pot, the larger the better. Cover with plenty of water.
3 Add 1 or 2 chopped carrots for sweetness, 1 or 2 onions or leeks, or any member of the onion family except garlic.
4 Add celery, fennel, or any similar salad vegetables that are available and season with bay leaves, peppercorns, thyme, a little rosemary, and handfuls of parsley.
5 Bring it to a boil and simmer for about 2 hours.
6 Strain off the bones and vegetables and discard them. Return the liquor to the pan and reduce it to about 2½ cups (600ml) in volume.
7 Cool the stock before storing it in the refrigerator or freezer. It will last for 3 days in the refrigerator.

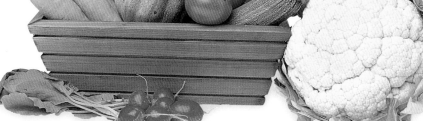

HOW TO COOK SOUPS

My recipe for homemade soup couldn't be simpler:

Ingredients
5 cups (1 liter) homemade stock (see p. 21)
1 or 2 potatoes
1 medium onion
Other ingredients as desired (see right)

Method
1 Place the stock in a large saucepan.
2 Chop up and add one or two potatoes. Add one peeled and diced medium-sized onion. Add any other ingredients as required.
3 Simmer the soup for 20–30 minutes. You can liquidize it if you want to make it thick and creamy.

Soups Once you have made your stock, it can be quickly transformed into a highly nutritious soup (see column, left). All the soups in my eating plan are potato-based, and for a good reason. Potatoes supply lots of carbohydrate and fiber. Leave the skins on because that's where all the minerals and vitamins are. You could also add one of the following suggestions to enliven your basic soup recipe.

Additional ingredients
• Carrots (diced or grated) and fresh coriander leaves.
• Leeks (2 or 3, omit the onion), 1 bay leaf, and parsley.
• 2 cups (225g) frozen peas and fresh mint.
• 1 cup (175g) brown or red lentils, 2 sticks of celery, black pepper, and 1 tsp (5ml) crushed coriander seeds.
• ⅔ cup (125g) grated cooked beets, seasoned with 1 tsp (5ml) ground cumin.
• ⅜ cup (50g) each of peas, cauliflower, and diced carrots, leeks, and rutabaga; black pepper, and parsley.

PORTIONS FOR FISH AND MEAT
When you follow my diet it is important that you eat correctly sized portions. The list below indicates the amounts of different fish, poultry, and meat you need to buy for each meal.

Fish
2oz (50g) anchovies in water
1 small herring or mackerel
6oz (175g) trout
4oz (125g) tuna in water
6oz (175g) whitefish (cod, haddock, coley, hake, plaice, sole, turbot)
1 medium-sized kipper
4oz (125g) monkfish
5oz (150g) salmon cutlet
4oz (125g) smoked salmon
6oz (175g) seafood (mussels, shrimp, scallops, crab)

Meat
2oz (50g) chicken livers
8oz (225g) turkey breast fillet
4oz (125g) smoked turkey
4oz (125g) calves' or lambs' liver
5oz (150g) chicken breasts
3oz (75g) boneless chicken
6oz (175g) rabbit, diced and boned

SALADS

I've put the salads into a special section because you can use them as a meal at any time. They are particularly nutritious and very filling, so any one of them will keep you going for a good two hours.

Mixed Salads

Mix together any amount of the following:

bean sprouts	cucumber	radicchio
carrot	endive	radish
celery	assorted lettuce	raw spinach
chicory	leaves	scallion
cress	green/red peppers	tomato

Dress with a little (2 teaspoons/10ml) of oil and vinegar dressing or 2 tablespoons (30ml) of very-low-fat plain yogurt dressing (see recipe, right) or 2 tablespoons (30ml) of rice vinegar. Alternatively, use one of the many low-fat dressings now available.

Broccoli Salad (serves two)

1lb (450g) broccoli, trimmed
2 sweet red peppers
For the tomato sauce:
1 clove garlic, crushed
½tbsp (7 ml)vegetable oil
½lb (225g) chopped tomatoes

1 Cook the broccoli until just tender, rinse with cold water, and drain well.
2 Slice the cold broccoli lengthwise into smaller pieces.
3 Grill the red peppers, turning them as they blacken. Wrap them in a clean cloth and let them cool for 10 minutes. Peel off the wrinkled skin and slice the peppers into thin strips, removing the seeds and the inner membranes.
4 Cook the crushed garlic in the oil until it just begins to brown, add the chopped tomatoes, and season with pepper. Simmer gently for 5 minutes or so.
5 Remove from the heat and liquidize or press through a sieve to make the sauce. Arrange the broccoli in a serving dish, pour the tomato sauce over it, and arrange the strips of red peppers on top. Allow to cool before eating.

YOGURT DRESSING

Ingredients
½ cup (150g) very-low-fat plain yogurt
1 tsp freshly ground black pepper, nutmeg, or cumin
½ tbsp (7ml) raspberry vinegar (or ordinary wine vinegar will do)
1 tbsp each chopped parsley, chives, leaf coriander
1 clove garlic, crushed
1 tbs (15ml) pine nuts or sesame seeds

Method
Place all the ingredients in a screw-top jar and shake firmly. This dressing will keep in the refrigerator for up to two days.

Eat well
Salads are light, nutritious, and quick to make. They are also high in fiber. Eat as much of them as you like.

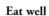

YOUR SHOPPING LIST

Use this list when you go shopping, but first work out at least the first few days of your seven-day eating plan and write down the specific ingredients for those dishes. Don't buy more than you need. Remember, fresh fish and organ meats are best eaten on the day they are bought.

	GROCERIES	BANNED FOODS
Fish and meat	Anchovies, herring, mackerel, kipper, monkfish, salmon, seafood (shrimp, mussels, scallops, crab), calves' or lambs' liver, chicken breast, turkey breasts, trout, tuna, whitefish (cod, haddock, coley, hake, plaice. sole, turbot), rabbit	*The following foods are strictly off-limits for the duration of the seven-day eating plan:*
Staples	Dried beans (aduki, chick peas, green flageolet, haricot, kidney), lentils, split peas, oatmeal, wholegrain (brown) rice, wild rice	• *Avocados*
Dairy	Cottage cheese, goat's or ewe's milk cheese, low-fat cheese, medium-sized eggs, milk (low-fat or skim), very-low-fat plain yogurt	• *Fried foods* • *Any red meat* • *Any refined or processed foods*
Vegetables	Asparagus, baby corn, beets, broccoli, cabbage, carrots, cauliflower, celeriac, corn, eggplant, garlic, green beans, leeks, okra, onions, parsnips, peas (frozen), potatoes (for baking and boiling), snow peas, spinach, zucchini	• *Any sauces, chutneys, and pickles*
Salad vegetables	Bean sprouts, celery, chicory, cucumber, fennel, lettuce, green/red peppers, radish, scallions, watercress, other salad leaves (e.g., endive, radicchio), tomatoes	• *All kinds of sugar, candy, and any jam, marmalade, or spread*
Fruit	Apples, apricots, bananas, berries (e.g., strawberries, raspberries, blueberries), dried fruit (e.g., apricots, prunes), grapefruit, lemons, limes, mango, melon, nectarines, oranges, papaya, peaches, pears, pineapple, other exotic fruit (e.g., guava, passion fruit)	• *Any canned foods in oil, syrup, or sauce*
Seasonings	Basil, bay leaves, chili pepper, red chili powder, chives, Chinese five spice, cilantro, coriander seeds, cumin, fennel seeds, fresh ginger root, marjoram, mint, mustard seed, nutmeg, parsley, pepper, black pepper, saffron, sage, tarragon, thyme, turmeric	
Other groceries	Herb teas, coffee, mustard (any as preferred), oil (olive/grapeseed/sunflower/safflower) for cooking and dressing, oil (olive/walnut/sesame) for flavoring, tomato juice, tomato puree, Tabasco, vinegar (wine/rice/raspberry), walnuts, hazelnuts	

THE SEVEN-DAY PLAN

If you think you have to starve yourself in order to lose weight, you are in for a pleasant surprise. On my diet you will probably eat more food than usual and still lose weight. Each day you will eat six balanced meals, choosing from a varied menu that caters both for meat-eaters and vegetarians. The seven-day plan also features tips on healthy eating, exercises to tone different parts of the body, and, best of all, every day there's a luxurious treat that you can give yourself. In a week's time, you will not only have lost weight, you will also have more energy and a greater zest for life.

THE PLAN

For the next seven days, I want you to stick only to the foods on the list I have given (see p. 24), and in order to keep your metabolism working in high gear it is important to eat six meals a day. Try to space them so that you don't go for more than two and a half hours without eating.

To make it easy, I have provided menu suggestions for each meal throughout the week and alternatives in case there is something you don't like. Once you have done the initial preparation for the six o'clock meals – the rice, dahl, and soup (see recipes, pp. 19–22) – only the lunch and dinner menus require any time and, depending on your situation, you may prefer to select quick and simple meals. Make sure that you drink at least two pints (one liter) of still water during each day. Try to drink a glass of water with every meal.

Drink for health
Water is refreshing and essential to your health. Drink plenty throughout the day to help flush out your system and reduce hunger pangs.

BREAKFAST

For breakfast each day, I really do recommend oatmeal, but if you would like an alternative, you can have up to two medium eggs during the week – either boiled, or for lunch as an omelette. Similarly, you can vary the pattern with a kipper occasionally. Make sure you have a piece of fruit as well, or if you prefer to have cereal, try an oats- or rice-based sugar-free one with fresh fruit chopped into it.

MIDMORNING SNACK

For your midmorning snack, I suggest another piece of fresh fruit – it needn't be just an apple if you take the trouble to stock up on some more unusual fruits before you start the diet. During the winter months you could treat yourself to mangoes and payayas and, during the summer, peaches and strawberries make wonderful snacks. If you like it, a 1oz (25g) slice of goat's or ewe's cheese works particularly well with a pear. A rice cake or low-fat yogurts are good ideas, too.

LUNCH

The lunch recipes are designed to cater for the office worker as well as for those of you who work at home. Many of the meals can be packaged easily so that they can travel with you. Others are more elaborate and might be more suitable for the weekend. All of them are appetizing enough to serve to the family or even to guests. In addition to eating the main course dish, have a dessert of fruit – perhaps some berries, a slice of pineapple, or choose from your fruit bowl – and, as always, drink plenty of still water.

MIDAFTERNOON SNACK

My family is fond of homemade plain oat cookies. They're not oatcakes; you make them with very little fat and no sugar and they're delicious (see recipe, p. 30). I suggest you have one of these, or a very low-fat yogurt or some more fruit for your midafternoon snack.

EARLY EVENING LIGHT MEAL

This is the time that most of us eat those high-calorie snacks that put on the weight. That's why it's so important to be well prepared with the right food for this meal, which is unprocessed carbohydrate in the form of hot soup, or three or four tablespoons of rice or dahl, or a mixture of both.

DINNER

I have given the dinner recipes in quantities suitable for two servings so that if you are eating with a partner or a friend, you can still make these recipes. If you are eating alone, just halve the ingredients. However, I think you'll find that your friends will be surprised at how tasty the meals on the eating plan are. I've included some ideas that may be new to you, such as tofu kebabs, and provided fish recipes, which are very nutritious and light; we should all eat fish more often. As you did for your lunch, choose your dessert from your fruit bowl. Remember to drink plenty of still water.

No fruit is forbidden
High in carbohydrate but low in calories, fruit is an ideal diet aid. Eat a piece of fruit whenever you feel hungry.

ONE-A-DAY SNACKS

If you are still hungry after eating all six meals in the eating plan, you may eat one of the following once a day:

- *1 whole piece of fruit*
- *1 boiled potato*
- *8 peeled shrimp*
- *1 slice of smoked salmon*
- *1 very-low-fat yogurt*
- *½ cup of soup*
- *1 small gelatin*
- *1 glass of tomato juice*

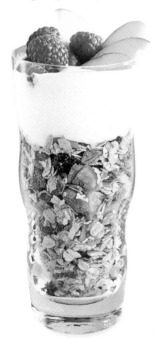

Deliciously healthy
This dessert is a healthy and tasty mix of sugar-free cereal, low-fat yogurt, and fresh fruit. It would also make an ideal breakfast meal.

MY BASIC GUIDELINES

These guidelines are the basic ideas that underpin my seven-day eating plan, and they will help you achieve a slimmer, fitter, and healthier lifestyle.

- Eat six times a day. Make each meal a ritual. Set the table and sit down to eat. Invite a friend to make it a social occasion.
- Remember that each dinner recipe serves two, unless otherwise specified.
- Take your food seriously and give it the benefit of your full attention. Chew your food thoroughly.
- Make breakfast a good meal by eating either hot or cold cereal, oatmeal for example, or a sugar-free brand of rice or oat bran flakes. Oats are particularly good for you because of their soluble fiber.
- Eat more fresh fruit, vegetables, and fish.
- Eat more beans and legumes. Plant protein is as good as animal protein! It isn't "second-class," as outdated theories suggested. You simply need to combine plant proteins to get all the amino acids you need.
- Eat smaller portions of red meat and fatty cheeses as a condiment to accompany green and root vegetables and rice, whole-wheat pasta, or potatoes.
- Eat more wholegrain products and less processed and refined foods (especially junk food).
- At every meal, eat the vegetables first and drink one or two glasses of water.
- Give up or reduce your intake of sugar and salt. Remove them from the dining table and stop using them in cooking. Be aware of the hidden sugar and salt in processed foods. Read food labels carefully and don't buy products that have added sugar or salt.
- If you get a craving for something sweet, try eating some unprocessed carbohydrate, such as fruit, raw vegetables or some cooked "bulk food" such as rice or dahl. Half an hour after eating this, your craving will be gone.
- Do moderate exercise for at least twenty minutes four times a week. This will keep your heart and lungs in good shape, your muscles toned, and your stamina reliable. Regular exercise has the added bonus of raising your metabolism so that you burn more calories – even when you're resting or asleep. Check with your doctor before starting an exercise plan.

DAY ONE

This is it. The beginning of your new diet plan. And today's menu has plenty of interesting flavors to kick-start your tastebuds so that you enjoy every mouthful.

Menu

BREAKFAST
Oatmeal (p. 19) with sliced dried apricots

MIDMORNING
A slice of whole-wheat bread or half a papaya with a squeeze of lemon or lime juice

LUNCH
Marinated Whitefish (p. 30)
or Orange and Kidney Bean Salad (p. 30)

MIDAFTERNOON
One plain oat cookie (p. 30), or a slice of whole-wheat bread, or half a mango with lemon juice

EARLY EVENING
A cup of hot soup (p. 22), or 3–4 tablespoons of rice (p. 19) or dahl (p. 20), or a mixture of both

DINNER
Oven-poached Chicken (p. 31)
or Tofu and Mixed Pepper Kebabs (p. 31)

EXERCISE OF THE DAY

The thighs are the biggest muscles in the body so they can burn up quite a few calories if they are exercised and toned.

Start exercising by concentrating on the thighs as you go about your day-to-day activities. Whenever you are walking, try to take bigger steps. Really stride out – this is obviously easier if you're wearing nonrestrictive clothing, such as pants. As a bonus, walking this way will also make you feel more positive and confident.

Aerobic activities, such as bicycling and running, also help burn fat from this area, so try to make them part of your exercise program. Specific muscle-toning exercises, such as the one shown below, can be done at any time – even while you're watching TV.

Start and end the exercise in this position

Tone your thighs
Stand straight with your feet hip-width apart and your arms in front of you. Bend your knees and extend your arms forward. Hold this position then slowly return to the upright position, working your thigh muscles. Repeat 10 times.

Stretch your arms out straight in front of you

Push your bottom out as if about to sit on a chair

RECIPES FOR DAY ONE

Marinated Whitefish

6oz (175g) fillet of whitefish
3 tsp lemon or lime juice
½ tsp fennel seeds, crushed
¼ red chili, finely chopped

1 Place all the ingredients in a dish and marinate them overnight in the refrigerator – no cooking necessary!
2 Serve the fish with a mixed salad tossed in 1 tsp french dressing (see p. 42), and ½ cup (125g) cooked wholegrain rice (see p. 19).

Orange and Kidney Bean Salad

1½ cups (75g) cooked kidney beans
1 large orange, peeled and cut into segments
2 sticks of celery, chopped
1 tbsp french dressing (p. 42) with wholegrain mustard
    and a dash of lemon juice
a large handful of iceberg lettuce
2oz (50g) hard cheese (goat or ewe preferably), sliced

1 Mix the beans, orange, and celery with the dressing and pile it onto a bed of lettuce.
2 Scatter the slices of cheese over the lettuce.
3 Serve it with ½ cup (125g) cooked wholegrain rice (see p. 19).

Plain Oat Cookies (Makes about 20)

1½ cups (175g) oatmeal
½ cup (50g) rolled oats
a pinch of baking soda
4 tbsp (50g) margarine
1 egg yolk

1 Mix together the dry ingredients and rub in the margarine until the mixture resembles dry breadcrumbs.
2 Add the egg yolk and mix to a firm dough, then knead lightly.
3 Roll out to a thickness of about ¼in (6mm) and cut into shapes; transfer to a greased cookie sheet.
4 Bake at 350°F/180°C for about 15 minutes or until darker in color. Store in an airtight tin.

Oven-poached Chicken

2 x 6oz (175g) chicken breasts (skin removed)
½ medium onion, sliced
6oz (175g) each of green beans, cabbage and celeriac,
cut into sticks
⅔ cup (150ml) stock (p. 21)

1 Arrange the chicken pieces in an ovenproof dish, scatter the green beans, cabbage, and celeriac over them, and pour in the stock.
2 Cover the dish and bake at 375°F/190°C for 30 minutes.
3 Serve with a baked potato.

Tofu and Mixed Pepper Kebabs

8oz (225g) firm tofu (bean curd), cut into
10 equal-sized cubes
1 tsp tomato puree
Tabasco
2 tbsp rice vinegar
1 tsp freshly grated ginger root
2 tsp sesame or olive oil
1 large green pepper
1 large sweet red pepper
1 large yellow pepper
5 closed-cup mushrooms

1 Make the marinade by mixing together the tomato puree, ginger root, and two or three drops of Tabasco, and rice vinegar.
2 Pour the marinade over the tofu cubes, cover, and leave to marinate for about an hour, turning the cubes from time to time to make sure the marinade impregnates each side.
3 Meanwhile cut each mushroom in half and cut the peppers into pieces the same size as the mushrooms.
4 When the tofu has marinated, push alternate pieces of tofu, pepper, and mushroom onto two long or four short kebab skewers, putting a piece of pepper on either side of each tofu cube. Brush the kebabs with oil.
5 Broil or barbecue, turning them frequently until the peppers start to brown and the tofu is cooked through.
6 Serve with 4oz (125g) cooked wholegrain rice (see p. 19) per person.

TIPS AND TREATS FOR DAY ONE

Tips   Take your food and mealtimes seriously. Make eating a separate and distinct part of your life, a familiar routine; in other words, sit down and concentrate on what you're eating.

• Avoid distractions: don't read the newspaper or watch television during mealtimes.

• Get into the habit of eating at the table; set the table properly before you begin your meal.

• Chew your food slowly and thoroughly, and drink plenty of water throughout the meal.

• Remember, your appetite control center takes a while to switch off the hunger signals. Do not stuff yourself, and stop eating as soon as you begin to feel full.

Treat for women   Your treat today is as much about setting aside a special time that is just for you, as how you choose to treat yourself. Although some women might feel guilty about pampering themselves, they'd all agree, however, that time spent on their face is rewarding, not only in terms of results but also in terms of their self-confidence.

A facial doesn't have to cost a lot because you can give yourself one at home, perhaps toward the end of the day as part of your winding-down activities. It's very relaxing to settle down to your chosen face treatment, even if it's only steaming your complexion over a bowl of hot water in which you've put two to three drops of lavender oil. A face pack is even more relaxing because you have to lie down with your eyes closed. On the other hand, a face massage can be invigorating.

Treat for men   Have you ever wondered what it's like to go to the barbershop and have a luxurious shave – the full works? Why not treat yourself to an old-fashioned razor shave, with hot and cold towels and skin lotions. You'll come out with your skin feeling as smooth as a baby's – and you'll look terrific, too.

Give your face a tonic
Try a face pack – they are excellent for cleansing and toning the skin because they stimulate the blood supply to the complexion. They also give you a chance to relax and pamper yourself a little.

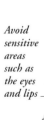

Avoid sensitive areas such as the eyes and lips

DAY TWO

You should have more energy from your healthy diet, and today it's time to start being more active – walk as much as you can. Get going if you seriously want to lose weight!

Menu

BREAKFAST
Oatmeal (p. 19) or half a grapefruit
and a grilled kipper

MIDMORNING
Fresh fruit – why not munch on an apple?

LUNCH
Stir-fried Turkey Breast (p. 34)
or Bean Salad (p. 34)

MIDAFTERNOON
An oat cookie (p. 30) or a banana

EARLY EVENING
Hot soup (p. 22), 2–4 tablespoons of dahl (p. 20),
or a cool glass of tomato juice

DINNER
Vegetable Hotpot (p. 35)
or Chicken, Salmon, or Trout Salad (p. 35)

EXERCISE OF THE DAY

From now on, wherever possible I want you to ignore elevators and escalators and walk up the stairs instead.

Don't rush into this if you are fairly unfit – start by walking up short flights and hold onto the handrail if you need support. As you feel fitter, you will be able to walk up without using the handrail. Next, try taking two steps at a time, using the handrail. Soon you'll be able to do two steps at a time without the help of the handrail. When you feel reasonably comfortable with that, run up the stairs, or escalators, two at a time! You can also do simple stepping and leg exercises at home (see below). All these activities will exercise your thighs and are good for your heart.

I also want you to walk whenever possible; this is an easy and stress-free way to do aerobic activity. Opt for a 15-minute walk rather than a five-minute drive, or get off the bus earlier.

Leg lifts
Lie on one side with one leg on top of the other. Raise the upper leg slowly to about 12in (30cm), hold it there, then lower it slowly. Repeat 10 times on each side to strengthen your thigh muscles.

Support your head on your hand

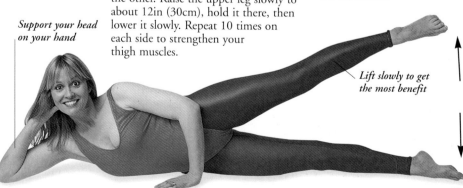

Lift slowly to get the most benefit

RECIPES FOR DAY TWO

Stir-fried Turkey Breast

2 tsp sesame or olive oil
8oz (225g) turkey breast fillet (fat removed)
4oz (125g) snow peas
4oz (125g) fennel, sliced
a pinch of Chinese five spice
scallions, chopped (optional)

1 Heat the oil in a wok or skillet.
2 Chop up the turkey fillet into thin strips.
3 Fry the turkey strips quickly over high heat.
4 Add the vegetables and spice, and stir continuously for two minutes; the vegetables should stay crunchy.
5 Scatter chopped scallions over the top.
6 Serve with two slices of whole-wheat bread or ½ cup (125g) cooked wholegrain rice (see p.19) per person, and ½lb (225g) baby corn.

Bean Salad

1¼ cups (175g) cooked weight of mixed dried beans
*   (soaked overnight)*
¼ cucumber, diced
1 heaped tsp chopped onion
black pepper to taste

Dressing

⅔ cup (150ml) very-low-fat yogurt
a dash of lemon juice
2 tsp parsley or chives, finely chopped

1 After soaking the beans overnight, rinse them and boil the beans without adding salt until they are tender. This may take at least 45 minutes.
2 Drain the beans thoroughly and put them in a serving dish. Add pepper if you like it. Leave them to cool.
3 Add the diced cucumber and onion and mix well with the beans.
4 Mix together the dressing ingredients and pour over the cooled bean salad, tossing well.
5 Accompany each serving with a slice of whole-wheat bread.

Vegetable Hotpot

2 tsp safflower or olive oil
1 onion, sliced
1 medium eggplant, diced
2 zucchini, sliced
½ cauliflower, cut into florets
2 tsp tomato puree
⅔ cup (150ml) stock (p. 21)
1 tsp dried basil
Tabasco and black pepper to taste
¾ lb (350g) potatoes, sliced
1 tbsp grated parmesan cheese

1 Heat 1 tsp oil in an ovenproof casserole dish.
2 Add the vegetables and fry for 2 minutes, then add the tomato puree, stock, and basil.
3 Season with Tabasco and black pepper and bring to a boil.
4 Arrange the potatoes on top, brush with 1 tsp oil, and bake at 375°F/190°C for 1 hour.
5 Ten minutes before serving, sprinkle the parmesan cheese on top.
6 Serve with 1½ cups (150g) whole-wheat pasta.

Chicken, Salmon, or Trout Salad

½ iceberg lettuce, chopped
a handful of rocket leaves
½ cucumber, peeled and diced
½ tbsp pine kernels
¼ lb (125g) cooked chicken, smoked salmon,
*   or trout*
french dressing (p. 42)
juice of half a lemon
black pepper to taste

1 Combine the salad ingredients and pine kernels, toss with the dressing, and divide between two plates.
2 Remove the skin from the chicken, or if using fish, remove the skin and bones from the fish, and slice it into strips.
3 Lay the chicken or fish on top of the salad, sprinkle sparingly with lemon juice, and season with pepper.
4 Serve with two slices of whole-wheat bread.

TIPS AND TREATS FOR DAY TWO

Tips You can gradually begin to cut down on your intake of meat by trying some of the following:

• Treat meat as a condiment: have four times as much vegetables as meat on your plate.

• Start by eating the vegetables and, if you begin to feel full, leave some meat on your plate.

• Choose some of the vegetarian options that I have suggested in the seven-day plan.

• When you have finished the seven-day plan, try not to eat red meat more than once a week.

• Try cooking with alternative protein foods, such as tofu, instead of meat.

• Try extending the meat or ground meat in meat pies and casseroles with the addition of some plant protein, such as lentils or Great Northern beans; these make up the core of many well-known delicious dishes, such as cassoulet from the south of France.

Treats Therapeutic massage is universally soothing and relaxing; it's fun if you can get someone else to do it for you, but you can also massage yourself. In some respects, self-massage is superior because you get the benefit twice – your body feels the calming pressure of your fingers but your fingers also feel the tranquilizing effect of stroking. Massage doesn't have to be vigorous – it's very sensuous just to run your fingers over your shoulders, neck, and arms; especially if you make the skin supple and slippery with aromatic oils. Useful essential oils for relieving stress are clary sage oil, lavender, and ylang ylang.

Alternatively, you could go have a full-body massage at your local beauty salon or leisure center. Or why not schedule yourself a full aromatherapy session?

Relax with a massage
Get your partner or a friend to massage your back and shoulders – this area is often tight as a result of stress. Use a relaxing massage oil such as lavender and don't forget to warm it before beginning.

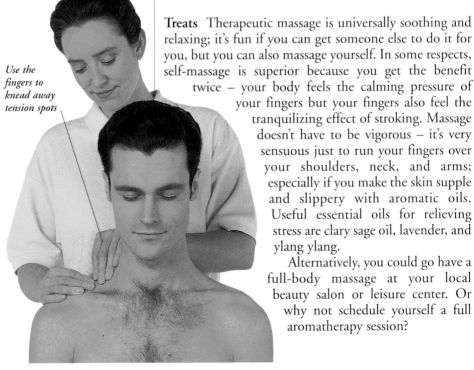

Use the fingers to knead away tension spots

DAY THREE

How are you feeling? Halfway through the week, you may be feeling a little lighter, more energetic, and possibly hungry. See my tips on how to cope with this.

Menu

BREAKFAST
Oatmeal (p. 19) sweetened with sliced prunes

MIDMORNING
A tangerine

LUNCH
Grilled Fish with Steamed Vegetables (p. 38)
or Mexican Green Beans (p. 38)

MIDAFTERNOON
A tomato or a rice cake

EARLY EVENING
A cup of soup (p. 22), 3–4 tablespoons of rice (p. 19),
or a baked potato

DINNER
Country Casserole (p. 39)
or Ratatouille (p. 39)

EXERCISE OF THE DAY

These exercises are designed to tone your stomach muscles and have a great effect on your waistline as well. They can be quite difficult to begin with, but soon become easy if you persist.

I want you to pull your stomach all the way in ten times. As that becomes easier, try holding it in for five seconds each time. This is such a simple exercise that you can do it anywhere, sitting at a desk, standing in a bus line, or even while you are walking, so make a point of doing it whenever you can. You'll be amazed at the results.

You can also begin by doing sit-ups, as shown below, in the morning or evening. It is a very small movement – just lift your head off the floor. Start by doing only a few and gradually increase the number as it becomes easier. If you do these exercises regularly, you'll be surprised by how soon you can do more.

Tummy tone-up
Lie on your back with your knees bent and feet flat on the floor. Put both hands at the back of your head. Lift your head toward your knees, pulling in your stomach muscles. Lower your head gently back to the floor.

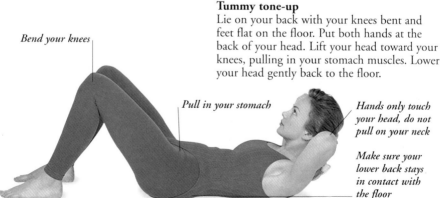

Bend your knees

Pull in your stomach

Hands only touch your head, do not pull on your neck

Make sure your lower back stays in contact with the floor

RECIPES FOR DAY THREE

Grilled Fish with Steamed Vegetables

½lb (225g) whitefish (cod, haddock, plaice, sole, monkfish)
1 tsp safflower or olive oil
½lb (225g) leeks, sliced
½lb (225g) zucchini, sliced
1½ cups (225g) green beans
wedges of lemon or lime, black pepper

1 Brush the fish with the oil.

2 Broil under a medium heat until it is cooked, turning once. Cooking time will vary depending on the thickness of your piece of fish. Check it frequently to make sure it doesn't dry out.

3 Meanwhile, place the sliced vegetables in a steamer over a pan of boiling water and steam until just cooked (do not let them get mushy).

4 Serve the fish with the wedges of lemon or lime, black pepper if liked, and the vegetables arranged around the fish. Accompany with ½ cup (125g) cooked wholegrain rice (p. 19) or a baked potato for each person.

Mexican Green Beans

1 tsp olive or sesame oil
1 cup (175g) Great Northern beans
(or use any green beans)
½ small onion, sliced
3 tbsp stock (p. 21)
½ red pepper, sliced
½ tsp tomato puree
pinch of chili powder or 1 fresh chili
(deseeded and sliced)

1 Heat the oil in a large skillet or a wok. (Watch out if you are using sesame oil, it burns very easily. If it does, it will taste bitter; throw it out and start again.)

2 Stir-fry the vegetables for two minutes.

3 Add the stock, tomato puree and chili powder (or sliced chili) and stir well.

4 Reduce the heat and simmer until almost all the liquid is absorbed.

5 Serve the beans with ½ cup (125g) cooked wholegrain rice (p. 19) per person.

Country Casserole

¾ lb (350g) cubed, boned rabbit (or chicken breasts)
1 clove garlic, crushed
2 sticks celery, chopped
3-4 medium carrots, chopped
1 medium onion, sliced
1⅓ cups (300ml) chicken stock (p. 21)
1 tsp french mustard
1 tsp tarragon
black pepper to taste

1 Arrange the meat in a casserole dish (chicken breasts can be substituted, if you prefer).
2 Add the vegetables.
3 Pour the chicken stock over the meat and vegetables, and add the mustard, tarragon, and black pepper.
4 Cover and cook for about 1½ hours at 375°F/190°C.
5 Serve with ½lb (225g) asparagus and leeks, lightly boiled or steamed, and a baked potato.

Ratatouille

(Makes approximately 8oz (225g) cooked weight per portion)

1⅓ cups (300ml) vegetable stock (p. 21)
⅜ cup (50g) chick peas, soaked overnight
1 clove garlic, crushed
1 tsp dried marjoram
1¼ cups (300ml) tomato juice
1lb (450g) tomatoes, quartered
1 medium eggplant, diced
2 zucchini, sliced
1 carrot, sliced
1 onion, sliced
1 green pepper, sliced

1 Put the vegetable stock into a pan.
2 Add the chick peas and bring to the boil.
3 Cover and simmer for 45 minutes, until the chick peas are tender.
4 Add all the other ingredients to the pan and simmer for a further 45 minutes.
5 Once the vegetables are cooked to your liking, serve with ¼ cup (25g) grated cheese on each portion, and a baked potato.

TIPS AND TREATS FOR DAY THREE

Tips If you feel hungry, you may be tempted to buy a sugary or fatty snack on impulse. A good way to stop yourself is to imagine how that cookie or bag of potato chips will end up in your body – perhaps as another ounce of fat on your thighs! What you are feeling may not be genuine hunger at all, particularly if you are sticking to my plan and eating six times a day. It could simply be a need for some oral gratification, and might be relieved by chewing a piece of sugarless gum.

However, if you do really feel hungry, eat some carbohydrate – but make certain it is unprocessed carbohydrate. Have something like a banana, half a baked potato, some rice or dahl, or, if you are at home, some homemade soup. If you eat one of these foods, half an hour after eating the hunger will have gone away.

Treats Hands are often neglected, so spending a half hour or so on pampering them is a real treat. Men, in particular, often neglect their hands, and can benefit from using moisturizer on their skin, and cleansing and filing their nails regularly.

1 Start as a manicurist would by soaking your hands in warm water to soften the cuticles and make cleaning easy. Dry your hands carefully.

2 Clean under the nails with an orange stick, file them into shape, then rub in rich hand cream.

3 Gently push back the cuticles with a cuticle stick. If you normally wear nail polish, remove the old polish with an acetone-free remover.

4 To achieve a professional look when applying nail polish, start with a base coat. Use a corrector pen to remove any smudges.

5 Apply two coats of color, allowing plenty of time for each layer to dry.

6 Reapply the top coat every third day; this manicure should last up to three weeks.

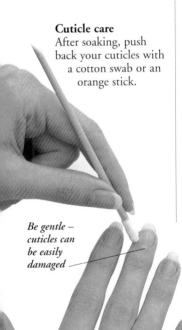

Cuticle care
After soaking, push back your cuticles with a cotton swab or an orange stick.

Be gentle – cuticles can be easily damaged

DAY FOUR

Now that you've become healthier, fitter, and more positive in your approach to eating and dieting, don't forget to give yourself a special treat – you've earned it!

Menu

BREAKFAST
A poached egg with a slice of whole-wheat bread followed by an orange

MIDMORNING
An oat cookie (p. 30) and a nectarine, if in season, or a slice of pineapple

LUNCH
Salad Niçoise with French Dressing (p. 42) or Stir-fried Tofu and Vegetables (p. 42)

MIDAFTERNOON
An apple, an oat cookie, or a slice of whole-wheat bread

EARLY EVENING
3–4 tablespoons of dahl (p. 20)

DINNER
Tandoori Chicken and Spicy Vegetables (p. 43) or Lentil and Potato Pie (p. 43)

Spinal stretch
Lie on your back with your knees raised and together. Slowly lower your knees to one side until they touch the floor and turn your head in the opposite direction. As you do this, visualize your entire spinal column being loosened. Repeat on the other side.

Turn your head in the opposite direction

Keep your feet and knees together

Spread your arms out to each side

EXERCISE OF THE DAY

Today there are two exercises. One is a lower back stretch (illustrated below), which is suitable for both men and women. It strengthens the lower back and tightens and trims the waist. The other, which is solely for women, tones the pelvic floor muscles.

Kegel exercise This is particularly important for women who have had children. It can stop you from developing incontinence in later life, or even a prolapse; both of which are fairly common. One bonus of this exercise is that it can improve your sexual enjoyment.

Method Pull up your pelvic floor slowly and hold for several seconds. The easiest way to learn how to contract these muscles is to try to stop the flow of urine when you go to the toilet. The muscles that you can feel are your pelvic floor muscles. This exercise may be difficult at first if you've neglected these muscles; practice when you go to the toilet and eventually you will be able to do it anywhere, any time.

41

FRENCH DRESSING

Ingredients
1 tsp safflower oil
1 tsp olive or other strong-flavored oil
1 tbsp lemon juice
1 tsp wine vinegar
½ teaspoon mustard
black pepper

1 Place all the ingredients in a screwtop jar.
2 Shake vigorously for one minute.
3 If not used immediately, this can be stored in the refrigerator for up to a week.

RECIPES FOR DAY FOUR

Salad Niçoise
a handful of crisp lettuce
¼ green pepper, sliced
½ cup (50g) green beans, cooked
1 stick of celery, chopped
1 tomato, sliced
1 tbsp onion, chopped
14-oz can (125g) tunafish in water, drained
2 anchovy fillets, soaked overnight in milk

1 Line a serving bowl with the lettuce.
2 Layer the vegetables on top of the lettuce.
3 Place the tunafish and anchovy fillets on top.
4 Make the french dressing (see column, left) and pour the dressing over the salad.
5 Accompany each serving with 1½ cups (150g) whole-wheat pasta, or a slice of whole-wheat bread.

Stir-fried Tofu and Vegetables
½ lb (225g) tofu (soft bean curd), cut into small cubes of about 1in (2cm)
4 cups (1 liter) vegetable stock (p. 21)
2 tsp sesame oil
1 scallion, finely sliced
1 cup (110g) bean sprouts
½ cup (50g) Chinese cabbage, finely shredded
2–3 brown cap or oyster mushrooms, sliced
a pinch of Chinese five spice
parsley (Chinese, if possible), chopped

1 Simmer the tofu cubes in vegetable stock for approximately five minutes. Drain and set them aside to keep warm.
2 Put the sesame oil into a large nonstick skillet or wok over a high heat, then add the scallions.
3 Stir-fry them for about three minutes, then add the bean sprouts, Chinese cabbage, and mushrooms.
4 Add the warm tofu cubes and a pinch of Chinese five spice and stir-fry for a further two minutes, taking care not to let the cubes break up.
5 Serve with 3–4 medium carrots, steamed and cut into strips. Sprinkle with chopped parsley.

Tandoori Chicken and Spicy Vegetables

2 x ¼lb (125g) chicken breast fillets
juice of one lemon

Spicy Vegetables
2 tsp sesame oil
¼lb (125g) baby new potatoes, parboiled
¼lb (125g) okra or eggplant
1½ cups (175g) cauliflower florets
1 medium zucchini, cut into sticks
2 tbsp chicken stock (p. 21)
½ tsp cumin seed
½ tsp black mustard seeds

1 Marinate the chicken in lemon juice for 10 minutes.
2 Add the yogurt marinade (see column, right) to the chicken and leave it for at least 2 hours or overnight.
3 Cook the chicken under the broiler for about 20 minutes, turning once and basting occasionally. (Tip: line the broiler tray with foil to make cleaning easy.)
4 While the chicken cooks, heat the oil in a large pan.
5 Stir-fry the vegetables; add the stock and seeds.
6 Once the liquid has been absorbed, serve the chicken and vegetables together, with ½ cup (125g) cooked wholegrain rice (p. 19) per person.

MARINADE

Ingredients
⅔ cup (150ml) low-fat plain yogurt
1 tsp tomato puree
1 clove garlic, crushed
a pinch each of ground chili, coriander, cumin, ginger, and pepper

1 Pour the yogurt into a bowl. Add the tomato puree and mix well.
2 Add the garlic and spices and continue stirring until thoroughly mixed.
3 Add to the meat.
4 You can make the marinade up to 12 hours in advance if you store it in the refrigerator.

Lentil and Potato Pie

½ cup (125g) brown lentils, presoaked
1¼ cups (225g) carrots, chopped
1 medium onion, sliced
1 clove garlic, crushed
1½ cups (300ml) stock (p. 21)
pinch of marjoram and black pepper
225g (8oz) potatoes, chopped and boiled
1 tbsp low-fat yogurt
1 tbsp scallion, chopped

1 Simmer the lentils, carrots, onion, and garlic in the stock until tender (this takes about 45 minutes).
2 Drain well, season with marjoram and pepper, and place in a pie dish.
3 Mash the potatoes with the yogurt, and cover the lentils. Sprinkle with the scallions.
4 Serve with a steamed vegetable such as cabbage.

TIPS AND TREATS FOR DAY FOUR

Tips If you eat salty food, your body retains more water, which adds to your weight and alters your shape. It's a good idea, therefore, to eat less salt, and to avoid salted snacks. In addition, try to eat more natural diuretics – these are foods that help you lose water. If you drink plenty of still water every day of the plan and keep natural diuretics on your menu, you will lose more weight.

The most easily available diuretics are:

• Parsley – a wonderful herb in its own right, and also a very convenient alternative to salt as a seasoning.

• Capsicums – (red, green, or yellow peppers) – as well as being a diuretic, they are also very rich in vitamin C (they have even more than citrus fruit).

• Asparagus – this is a delicious treat and a powerful diuretic. You may notice the effect before the meal ends!

• Real coffee – have a cup of this in the morning if you like it. But don't have too much or drink it late at night because it can make you irritable and you'll sleep less well.

Treat Today's treat is to take advantage of your local health club for a day. Go with your partner or with a friend to make it more enjoyable. You might have a strenuous workout or alternatively have a day of luxury and relaxation.

There are bound to be saunas, steam rooms, or somewhere just to lie back and relax, so take a book, magazine, or your personal stereo with you. Even just a change of scene will make a real treat. You may find that a facial and massage are also available and both will give you a boost. You'll feel really spoiled if you have someone else pamper you, and you may learn a few tricks and perhaps treat yourself to a few luxury beauty or sports products.

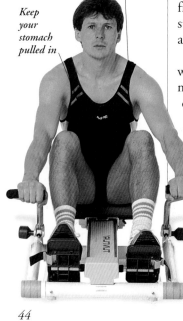

Wear lightweight clothes when exercising to avoid becoming overheated

Keep your stomach pulled in

Exercising at the gym
If you haven't exercised for some time, take it easy at first. An instructor will show you how to use the equipment and you will soon build stamina and confidence.

DAY FIVE

The seven-day plan, with its emphasis on healthy food and exercise, means that you're on the way to looking younger, revitalized, and radiant with health. Keep going!

Menu

BREAKFAST
Brown Rice Breakfast Dish (p. 46)

MIDMORNING
24 (½ cup) blackberries, blueberries, or raspberries

LUNCH
Seafood Salad (p. 46) or Spanish Omelette (p. 46)

MIDAFTERNOON
A pear with, if you like, a slice of goat or ewe cheese

EARLY EVENING
3–4 tablespoons of rice (p. 19) or dahl (p. 20), or one very-low-fat yogurt

DINNER
Stuffed Peppers, Tomatoes, or Eggplant (p. 47), or Steamed Mussels (p. 47)

Swing and stretch
With your arms extended, swing your body to one side, then the other. Repeat 20 times. This exercise trims the waist and relaxes the neck muscles.

As you swing, twist your hips slightly

Keep your feet about 2ft (50cm) apart

EXERCISE OF THE DAY

Improving your posture can instantly make you look slimmer. If you have been doing the suggested exercises for the last four days, you have probably already improved your posture, but now I want you to think about it more specifically.

Don't look down as you walk around, since this encourages droopy shoulders or even a dowager's hump in later life. It's also bad for your breathing, your digestion, and your back. Hold your head up and keep your shoulders back – although not too stiffly!

Try standing correctly in front of a mirror; you should find that you look taller, your silhouette has improved, and your clothes fit better. What's more, you will look more confident. Research shows that muggers will be less inclined to pick on you because you will look and feel more confident and also assertive.

Try to stretch every day, especially before you begin any exercise routine. In addition to improving your posture, stretching exercises will help to keep you supple and also help prevent injury.

45

OPTIONAL BREAKFAST INGREDIENTS

Add any of the following to your cooked rice:

- *sesame or sunflower seeds*

- *ground almonds*

- *3 tbsp (25g) finely grated carrot*

- *2 tbsp (25g) fruit puree (apricot, apple, pear)*

- *1 tsp light tahini (for a creamy texture and flavor)*

RECIPES FOR DAY FIVE

Brown Rice Breakfast Dish

½ cup (125g) cooked, short-grain brown rice
½ cup (100ml) water or water and juice of soaked, dried fruit

1 Combine all the ingredients of your choice (see column, left) in a saucepan, except for the fruit puree.
2 Stir over a medium heat, bring to a boil, then reduce the heat, cover, and simmer for five minutes.
3 Add the fruit puree, if using, just before serving.

Seafood Salad

6oz (175g) mixed steamed seafood (mussels, clams, shrimp, scallops, crab)
1 small carrot, cut into ribbons with vegetable peeler
1 scallion, shredded
lemon juice and 1 tsp olive oil

1 Place the seafood in a bowl.
2 Scatter the carrot and onion over the seafood.
3 Flavor sparingly with the lemon juice and olive oil.
4 Serve with one slice of wholemeal bread per serving.

Spanish Omelette

2 tsp olive oil
½ small onion, finely chopped
1 small sweet red pepper, sliced thinly
4 medium eggs
4 medium-sized potatoes, peeled, cut into ½-in (1-cm) cubes and boiled until tender, but not soft
½ cup (110g) cooked peas
black pepper to taste and parsley, finely chopped

1 Heat the olive oil in a heavy-bottomed, nonstick skillet and sweat the onion and pepper for a few minutes until the onion is translucent but not brown.
2 Set the onion and pepper mixture aside to keep warm.
3 Crack the eggs into a small bowl, beat them, and season with black pepper.
4 Pour the eggs into the pan. Cook over a medium heat until the bottom of the omelette has set.
5 Scatter all the vegetables evenly over the omelette.

6 Place the skillet under a hot broiler until the top of
the omelette is cooked through but not too brown.
7 Sprinkle the parsley on top of the omelette.
8 Serve with one slice of whole-wheat bread per serving
and, if you want, a mixed salad.

Stuffed Peppers, Tomatoes, or Eggplant

1 or 2 green peppers or large tomatoes,
or 1 eggplant, for each person

Stuffing

1 cup (225g) cooked brown rice
¾ cup (75g) frozen peas and sweetcorn
½ small onion, finely chopped
1 heaping tbsp mixed fresh herbs, chopped
black pepper to taste
¾ cup (150ml) tomato juice

1 Hollow out the vegetables.
2 Mix together all the stuffing ingredients, moisten
them with tomato juice, and stuff the mixture into the
vegetable shells. Arrange the shells in an ovenproof dish.
3 Pour in enough water to cover the bottom of the
dish. Cover and bake for 45 minutes to 1 hour at
375°F/190°C.
4 Serve with a baked potato.

Steamed Mussels

1½lb (700g) fresh mussels
¾ cup (150ml) vegetable or fish stock (p. 21)
1 onion, finely chopped
1 cup (125g) each bean sprouts, snow peas, green beans
1 heaped tbsp parsley, chopped

1 Clean and debeard the mussels, discarding any that
are not firmly shut.
2 Bring the stock and onion to a boil.
3 Add the mussels, cover, and simmer for three minutes,
giving the pan an occasional shake.
4 Remove from the heat, and allow to stand for two
minutes. Then remove the mussels from the pot, reject
any that have not opened, and keep them warm.
5 Cook the vegetables, to taste, in the mussel liquor.
6 Garnish with parsley and serve with a baked potato.

TIPS AND TREATS FOR DAY FIVE

Tips   Never let yourself get too hungry while on the seven-day eating plan or afterward. If you feel genuinely hungry, it's much better to bring your meal forward a little, because if you become ravenous, you might wolf down more food than you actually need. It is important to eat slowly until you are comfortably full.

Don't forget to drink lots of pure water to cleanse your body of toxins and waste products. Avoid carbonated drinks and some fruit juices, which can be high in sugar.

Treat   Give yourself a pedicure today so that you'll feel really pampered. It's so easy and the results will make your feet look fabulous. Try to make it a weekly event for long-term results.

1 Start with a short soak for about ten minutes to soften the hard skin – then it's easier to remove.

2 Dry your feet carefully with a warm towel. Clip your toenails and file smooth any rough corners.

3 Rub the soles with a cream body exfoliant to get rid of any loose dead skin, or rub with a wet pumice stone.

4 Wash off the exfoliant and dry the feet.

5 Treat your feet to rich foot or body cream; massage it in thoroughly.

6 If you like to wear nail polish, clean your toenails with an acetone-free polish remover and paint your toenails as described on day three (see p. 40). Go mad with color – while your fingernails can be sober, your toenails could be an extravagant gold, silver, navy-blue, or green.

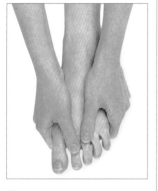

Foot care
For some, having a foot massage is the nearest thing to pure pleasure. A relaxed pair of feet will also help your posture and improve the way you walk. Work cream into the entire foot with circular movements.

DAY SIX

Your treat today suggests that you do something different because there's a lot to be said for getting out of your normal routine – it's a great life-enhancer – enjoy!

Menu

BREAKFAST
Oatmeal (p. 19) with an apple,
or one boiled egg and an orange

MIDMORNING
Two basic biscuits (p. 50)

LUNCH
Chicken or Monkfish Kebabs (p. 50)
or Cottage Cheese and Walnut Salad (p. 50)

MIDAFTERNOON
A cup of homemade soup (p. 22) or
a slice of melon

EARLY EVENING
3–4 tablespoons rice (p. 19) or dahl (p. 20)

DINNER
Bean and Vegetable Casserole (p. 51)
or Turkey Florentine (p. 51)

EXERCISE OF THE DAY

The following stretching exercises are for your back, upper arms, and, particularly, for your pectoral muscles on the front of your chest. For women, they may help raise the bust slightly as well.

For the first stretch, reach up your back as far as you can with one hand and meet it with the other coming over your shoulder. Now stretch down and try to clasp your hands together. Feel the muscles stretching in your chest and shoulders. Don't worry if you can't make your fingers meet at first, keep trying and it will become easier because all the time you are loosening your upper body. Try to do this five times a day, three or four times a week to begin with.

Another upper body stretch is easier. Put the palms of your hands together behind your back with the fingers pointing upward. Start off gradually and see how far you can get up your back. Don't do too much at first; if it hurts, stop. Do this ten times every day.

Push-ups
Kneel down, placing your hands flat on the floor, shoulder-width apart. Breathe in and lower yourself until your chin is close to the floor. Lift your body by straightening your arms. (Men can rest on their toes, not their knees).

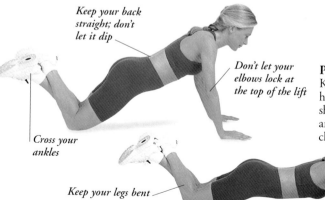

Keep your back straight; don't let it dip

Don't let your elbows lock at the top of the lift

Cross your ankles

Keep your legs bent

MONKFISH MARINADE

Ingredients
4 tsp orange juice
1 tsp coriander seeds

1 Crush the coriander seeds.
2 Mix together the orange juice and crushed coriander seeds.
3 Pour the marinade over the fish and marinate for about two hours.

RECIPES FOR DAY SIX

Basic Biscuits

1⅔ cups (175g) mixed bean flours
2 tbsp (25g) margarine or oil
1½–2½ tbsp (50–75ml) water
2 tbsp (25g) sesame seed meal (optional)
2 tsp baking powder (optional)

1 Mix together all the ingredients thoroughly.
2 Drop spoonfuls onto a lightly greased baking sheet.
3 Bake the biscuits at 325°F/170°C for 15 minutes. When cooled, store in an airtight tin.

Chicken Kebabs

3oz (75g) boneless chicken, cut into cubes
2oz (50g) chicken livers
¼ each of green, red, and yellow peppers
1 tsp safflower oil

Monkfish Kebabs

¼lb (125g) monkfish, cut into strips
6 cherry tomatoes
thick slices of onion
1 tsp safflower oil

1 If you are using monkfish, marinate the strips for two hours (see column, left).
2 Arrange kebabs on skewers, alternating meat or fish and vegetables in a colorful way.
3 Lightly brush them with oil and place under a hot broiler or over a barbeque.
4 Cook the kebabs for 10 minutes, turning occasionally.
5 Serve with a mixed salad and ½ cup (125g) cooked wholegrain rice (p. 19) per person.

Cottage Cheese and Walnut Salad

a large handful of endive
½ apple and ½ onion, sliced
½ head of chicory
½ cup (125g) low-fat cottage cheese
1 tbsp walnuts, chopped
1 tsp mint and ½ tsp walnut oil

1 Arrange the endive, apple and onion slices, chicory, and cottage cheese attractively on a plate.
2 Scatter with the walnuts and mint.
3 Trickle the oil over or toss it all together if preferred.
4 Serve with ¾ cup (75g) warm (not hot) whole-wheat pasta (per person).

Bean and Vegetable Casserole

1¼ cups (225g) dried green flageolet beans,
*   soaked overnight*
6⅓ cups (1.5 liters) vegetable stock (p. 21)
1 bay leaf
1 onion, chopped
1 large leek, cleaned and sliced
2 zucchini, chopped
1 tsp basil and ½ tsp each marjoram and oregano
black pepper to taste

1 Place the soaked beans, 4½ cups (1 liter) of the vegetable stock, and the bay leaf in a pan. Cover and simmer until the beans are tender but not mushy; this takes about two hours.
2 Transfer the cooked beans to a casserole dish with the onion, leek, and zucchini.
3 Pour in the remaining stock and the herbs and season with black pepper to taste.
4 Place the dish in the oven at 350°F/180°C for about 45 minutes, or until the vegetables are cooked.
5 Serve with two slices of whole-wheat bread.

Turkey Florentine

1½lb (700g) leaf spinach
nutmeg, black pepper, and 1 clove garlic
6 tomatoes, sliced
2 x 6oz (175g) turkey breast fillets (skin removed)

1 Cook the spinach until just wilting, squeeze out the excess liquid, chop it, and season with nutmeg, black pepper, and a crushed clove of garlic.
2 Spread the spinach on the bottom of a baking dish.
3 Arrange the sliced tomato over the spinach and place the turkey breasts on top.
4 Cover and bake at 375°F/190°C for 30 minutes.
5 Serve with a baked potato.

TIPS AND TREATS FOR DAY SIX

Tip You may have heard people say, "Don't eat protein with carbohydrate" and wondered what they meant. Well, there is something in this and it has to do with carbohydrate cravings. If you get the occasional urge to binge on sugary things, you are probably a carbohydrate craver. I explain the scientific theory behind the term on page 63; suffice it to say that when you are trying to satisfy this craving, you will get better results if you don't mix lots of protein with your unprocessed carbohydrate. Follow this advice and you will probably feel better more quickly and the craving will go away and stay away for several hours.

Treats These days, few of us have time for a really relaxed shopping trip, so your treat today is that you are going to take a whole day looking around the stores.

Give yourself plenty of time, including a stop at a favorite cafe for a cup of tea or coffee (without milk!). You could even have lunch if you choose the venue carefully to fit in with your daily plan, especially if you have a good friend to accompany you, who can make sure you stick to your diet.

Plan your route, don't be deterred or distracted, and be single-minded about your goals. Wear clothes with zippers or elastic for easy dressing and undressing when trying on garments.

If shopping doesn't appeal, however, or if you want to wait until you've finished the seven-day plan before you try on new clothes, do something that isn't normally part of your typical day. For example, you could go to a jazz club or an art exhibition, see an avant-garde play or a concert – the main idea is to do something that will broaden your horizons and make you feel good.

DAY SEVEN

You've reached the end of your seven-day diet plan – you should be feeling and looking great. Tomorrow you can weigh yourself and give yourself a huge pat on the back.

Menu

BREAKFAST
A bowl of oatmeal (p. 19) with one piece of melon sliced into it

MIDMORNING
One plain oat cookie (p. 30) or one basic biscuit (p. 50)

LUNCH
Spiced Liver Stir-fry (p. 54) or Rice and Lentil Salad (p. 54)

MIDAFTERNOON
A medium-sized apple or a rice cake

EARLY EVENING
3–4 tablespoons of dahl (p. 20)

DINNER
Poached Salmon Cutlets (p. 55) and Cucumber Salad (p. 55) or Edam Coleslaw (p. 55)

EXERCISE OF THE DAY

There are two exercises today, which are aimed at helping to tone your back, hips, and bottom.

For the first exercise, kneel on the floor and support your weight on your forearms. Lift each leg as shown below – the movement is slow.

Second, lie down on your back with your knees raised and your hands by your side. Now lift your buttocks off the floor as high as you can. Keep them firmly clenched, count to five, then lower them slowly. Repeat five times. This exercise concentrates on the bottom – do it every day.

Buttock toning
Kneel down with your weight on your forearms. Keep your back straight. Lift one leg and straighten it behind you. Raise it up and down slowly, holding your head up. Repeat this ten times with each leg.

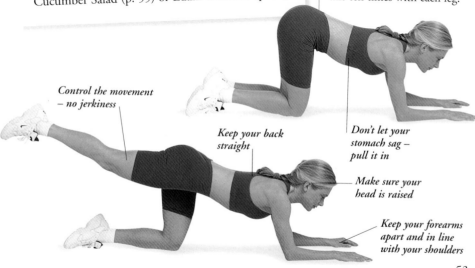

Control the movement – no jerkiness

Keep your back straight

Don't let your stomach sag – pull it in

Make sure your head is raised

Keep your forearms apart and in line with your shoulders

LIVER MARINADE

Ingredients
1 tbsp raspberry or wine
  vinegar
1 tbsp safflower oil
1 tsp ground cumin
½ tsp ground coriander
Tabasco to taste

1 Mix together all the marinade ingredients in a screw-top jar.
2 Shake vigorously to combine them well.
3 Pour the marinade over the liver, leave it for two hours.
4 Drain the liver before stir-frying it.

RECIPES FOR DAY SEVEN

Spiced Liver Stir-fry

2 tsp sesame or olive oil
½ cup (50g) carrots
½ cup (50g) bean sprouts
½ cup (50g) zucchini
½ cup (50g) green beans
2 tbsp chicken stock (p. 21)
2½oz (65g) lambs' or calves' liver, cut into strips

1 Marinate the lambs' or calves' liver (see column, left) for two hours.
2 Heat the oil in a skillet or wok and stir-fry the vegetables over a high heat for a few minutes.
3 Add the marinated liver and stir-fry for a further 3 or 4 minutes.
4 Serve with ½ cup (125g) cooked wholegrain rice (p. 19) per person.

Rice and Lentil Salad

½ cup (125g) rice
½ cup (125g) brown or green lentils
4 tomatoes, peeled and chopped
1 bunch scallions, chopped
1 small bunch coriander, washed and chopped
⅔ cup (150ml) low-fat plain yogurt
juice of ½ lemon
black pepper to taste

1 Cook the rice and lentils in boiling water in separate pans. Do not use salt when cooking the lentils – this hardens them.
2 Drain them both, mix together, and allow to cool.
3 Stir in the tomatoes, scallions, coriander, and the yogurt mixed with the lemon juice.
4 Season with pepper and serve.
5 If fresh coriander is unavailable, use 2 teaspoons of ground coriander seeds instead. Roast the seeds in a hot, dry skillet, allow to cool, and then crush them with a pestle and mortar or in an electric grinder. The taste will be different, but just as delicious.
6 Serve it with a green salad.

Poached Salmon Cutlets

2 x 5oz (150g) salmon cutlets

Court bouillon

3 cups (600ml) water
1 carrot and 1 onion, diced
1 stick celery, chopped
1 tsp wine vinegar or lemon juice
a handful of parsley, chopped
6 peppercorns

1 Combine all the ingredients for the *court bouillon* and heat gently.
2 Place the cutlets in a pan. Cover them with the warm *court bouillon* and bring to a simmer – do not boil.
3 Once the liquor is visibly swirling, leave to cook for about five minutes, then test the cutlets with a knife.
4 Serve with Cucumber Salad (see below) and ½ cup (125g) cooked wholegrain rice (p. 19) or a baked potato.

Cucumber Salad

half a cucumber, diced
1 clove garlic, crushed
2 tsp mint, chopped
⅔ cup (150ml) low-fat plain yogurt
black pepper to taste

1 Place the cucumber, garlic, and mint in a small bowl.
2 Pour the yogurt over and mix well. Season to taste.
3 This also makes a healthy snack or lunch when served with a slice of whole-wheat bread.

Edam Coleslaw

¼lb (125g) Edam cheese, cut into thin strips
½ cup (50g) white cabbage, shredded
1 carrot, grated
1 tsp grated onion
1 tbsp pine kernels
½ dessert apple, peeled and chopped
black pepper to taste
2 tbsp yogurt dressing (p. 23)

1 Mix together the first seven ingredients in a bowl.
2 Toss well with the yogurt dressing.
3 Serve with two slices of whole-wheat bread.

TIPS AND TREATS FOR DAY SEVEN

Tips If you really enjoy the taste of salt and are missing it, there are other ingredients that will give your food that extra flavor. Here are some replacements:

• You can release natural sodium from a host of fragrant herbs simply by sweating them gently over a low heat with a finely chopped onion and a teaspoon of oil. Keep the lid on the pan so the flavors can't escape, shaking the pan occasionally.

• Use a large quantity of fresh herbs in your cooking – coriander is particularly strong and dill has a delicious, sweet taste.

• For a real taste explosion, try chopping one or two fresh green or red chilies (the mild ones, not the fiery ones) into any cooked dish, but be sure to warn your fellow diners. When preparing them, take out the seeds first and afterward be careful to wash your hands before touching your eyes.

Treat A new hairstyle is the ultimate treat for many women, not just because a woman's hair should be her crowning glory but because it can take years off your age. And it's exactly the same for men.

A good hairstyle can reveal your best facial features, and it can also bring you up-to-date with the latest looks – this always boosts your self-esteem. Just before you go, discover which hairdressers are doing what by skimming the latest magazines or talking to your friends. Take a picture with you for guidance and discuss what you want with the stylist before she or he begins. Having a new color rinse, streaking, or tips is the ultimate indulgence, but it's usually worth it.

CHAPTER

NUTRITION

Today, it's possible to eat a well-balanced diet containing
all our essential nutrients cheaply and easily. The most
important requirement is that you choose from the widest
possible spectrum of foods. Try always to eat as much fresh
and, preferably, uncooked foods as possible for maximum
nutritional benefit. Fruit, vegetables, and salads should be
the mainstays of your diet, closely followed by unprocessed
carbohydrate such as whole-wheat bread, brown rice,
potatoes (not fried), pasta, cereals, and legumes.
Protein is essential but eat it in the form of fish, poultry,
and low-fat dairy products, rather than red meat. Animal
fat should be avoided but fish oils and plant oils contain
essential fatty acids and help protect the heart.

THE CHANGING PATTERN OF DIET AND DISEASE

Several million years ago, when our ancestors were scratching out a living on the African plains, their diet consisted largely of fruit, nuts, and vegetables. Whether as hunters or scavengers, they ate meat only now and then and were, for the most part, gatherers. Our teeth testify to our ancestors' omnivorous eating habits and so, less obviously, does our digestive system.

It was a menu of fresh fruit, seeds, nuts, and roots when available, topped up with the occasional blow-out of meat. Unlike us, our ancestors probably spent a good deal of their time munching, since vegetation is not a rich source of calories.

Now the world is a very different place. In the US, hunger is no longer such a widespread problem: in fact, quite the opposite. Today, the Western world has replaced malnutrition due to insufficiency with malnutrition and disease caused by excess or bad eating habits.

Obesity first became noticeable among the upper classes in the nineteenth century but the most dramatic transition in our national eating habits came after World War II. The post-war boom in agriculture saw a massive increase in the production and consumption of meat and dairy products. Ironically, the period of food rationing had produced a diet that was remarkably beneficial but all the benefit vanished as people gratefully switched away from bulky vegetable meals to more calorie-rich and fatty foods.

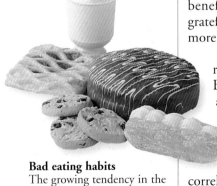

Bad eating habits
The growing tendency in the West to eat foods consisting of refined carbohydrate and saturated fats has caused an increase in the incidence of obesity and heart disease.

Now certain regions of the United States have reasonable claim to the title of Heart Attack Blackspot of the World. The incidence of coronary artery disease, obesity, hypertension, diabetes, and all the "diseases of affluence and overeating" (diverticular disease, cancer of the colon, constipation, hemorrhoids, gallstones, to name a few) has risen in the US in direct correlation with our change to a more refined, calorie-rich, and fatty diet.

How can we be sure that our diet is to blame for these twentieth-century diseases? After all, hardly anything has remained the same in our lives since the war. Evidence gathered from the study of other countries' eating habits and their patterns of disease can be quite persuasive. Certainly, although we are all one species, research shows that patterns of diet and disease vary dramatically from one culture to another.

The traditional diet of one of the last remaining hunters, the Eskimo, consists largely of meat, because agriculture is rather difficult on the ice-floes. Yet, despite a lifetime of eating flesh and blubber, the incidence of heart attacks is very low. The difference may well be due to the source of the flesh: the Eskimo diet consists mainly of fish, not animal meat.

In rural Africa and South America, heart disease is also rare but, as Westernization proceeds, so the incidence increases. The same has happened in Japan. Twenty-five years ago the Japanese diet of mainly fish and vegetables kept the nation virtually heart attack-free. But since then we've seen the effect of them switching to a Western diet – the incidence of heart attacks is approaching the level of that in the West.

Perhaps the most compelling evidence comes when we compare disease rates in other developed countries. Finland used to have the highest death rate from coronary artery disease until they changed their eating habits as a nation and stopped eating full-fat dairy products such as milk, butter, and cheese. Similarly, across the US and Western Europe, people have adjusted their diets and the incidence of heart disease has dropped. But the change has been slow, and some countries, furthermore, have been led astray by bad advice, especially in the vexed area of heart-healthy eating (see p. 64).

For years, a high-protein diet, falsely attributed to the Mayo Clinic, gathered many adherents. On this diet, all kinds of red meat, smoked meat, bacon, ham, and pork were allowed, as were eggs. It took years to undo the harm that this diet did, with its dangerous emphasis on high levels of animal fat, salty red meats, and high-cholesterol eggs. But it was only when we had incontrovertible proof that high animal fat intake led to high cholesterol levels, which in turn predisposed us to heart disease, that the harm could be undone. It took us even longer to find out that not all fats were bad, but that unsaturated fats and fish oils actually helped prevent heart disease.

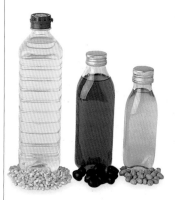

Are fats harmful?
Not all fats are bad. Your diet should include unsaturated fats, such as those found in oily fish and olive oil, which help keep your heart healthy.

FATS AND CHOLESTEROL

In recent years there has been increasing concern over the role of saturated fat in the development of coronary artery disease.

The concern revolves around the different way saturated and unsaturated fats are transported in the bloodstream. Since fats (lipids) are insoluble in water, in order to get around the bloodstream they have to be combined with protein, making a lipoprotein. But there is a third component in this transport system: cholesterol.

There has been a great deal of confusion and premature judgment on the culpability of cholesterol in coronary artery disease. Much of this arises from its close association with fat in lipoproteins. When lipids are traveling to or from adipose tissue (stores of fat) or muscle, they have, relatively speaking, a very low density. These lipoproteins are therefore called very low-density lipoproteins. After the fatty part has been delivered, its place is taken by cholesterol in the blood and it becomes a low-density lipoprotein.

Finally, the transport system can load up with extra protein for some journeys, making high-density lipoprotein. Dangerous cholesterol deposits are derived from low-density lipoprotein carriers (LDLs). If your LDL level is high, your risk of a heart attack is raised.

NUTRITION: FACT AND FICTION

As far as the body is concerned, there are three major categories of food: fats, proteins, and carbohydrates. Unfortunately, part of the confusion over what constitutes a good diet has arisen precisely because nutritionists have insisted on seeing a food as a source of protein or starch, rather than as a source of nutrition with a wide variety of useful and not so useful components. One example is liver, which is an excellent source of protein, vitamins, and minerals but is also high in cholesterol, so it is best to eat it only occasionally. To take another example, until recently cheese was recognized as a valuable source of protein. Now, however, many people recognize it as a potential source of undesirably high levels of saturated fat.

Like all animal products, dairy or meat, cheese has enjoyed an unjustifiably high level of prestige because the powerful food lobby of farmers, manufacturers, and retailers has promoted its own interests. One unfortunate spin-off of this promotion of cheese, whole milk, eggs, and meat as staple items of our diet has been the entirely erroneous idea that somehow plant proteins are inferior to animal proteins. All proteins are made of the same component parts, some 22 different amino acids. Neither plants nor animals nor the human digestive system makes any distinction between animal or plant-derived amino acids. They can't because the amino acids are identical.

PROTEIN

Enzymes, antibodies, muscle, skin, cartilage, blood, and other tissues are all largely composed of protein. Since all the body's proteins are continually broken down into amino acids and rebuilt in an inefficient way, the body needs a daily regular supplement of protein. Eight of the 22 amino acids cannot be made in the body. These eight are called "essential" amino acids and a good diet must include them. In general, animal products tend to have a more even spread of the different amino acids and more of the essential ones, whereas plants may have high concentrations of just a few. For instance, cereals tend to be low in lysine, one of the essential amino acids, but happily beans and legumes are rich in lysine. A vegetarian diet must therefore contain a very wide variety of vegetable foods to provide all the amino acids, whereas only a little meat will provide the same cover. Red meat, however, contains animal fat, and now that high levels of saturated fats are so strongly implicated in heart disease we must eat more plant protein. That is why my eating plan, with its emphasis on unprocessed carbohydrates, fruit, vegetables, and legumes, with red meat added only as a condiment, will help keep your heart healthy.

FATS

Made from fatty acids, fats provide the body with energy in its most concentrated form. Fatty acids are known as saturated or unsaturated depending on how "saturated" they are with hydrogen atoms. Saturated fatty acids tend to be harder, and solid at room temperature. Polyunsaturates remain liquid at room temperature. With the exception of coconut and palm oils, almost all plant-derived oils are polyunsaturated or monounsaturated.

The principal sources of saturated fat are animal products: milk, cheese, butter, and meat. Keep your fat intake down by eating these foods rarely, or only those with a lower fat content. Better still, avoid red meat and eat fowl, fish, and legumes instead. Just as some amino acids cannot be made by the body, so certain fatty acids are essential to the diet; these are all polyunsaturates. One in particular, linoleic acid, is the precursor of arachidonic acid, which is found in cell membranes and prostaglandins, hormones that help regulate many vital functions of the body. Everyone's diet should include such foods as oily fish, vegetable oils, and nuts, all of which contain these essential fatty acids.

CARBOHYDRATES, SUGAR, AND FIBER

The word carbohydrate can mean sugar, starch, or cellulose, depending on context. Whereas fat is reasonably easy to recognize in food, the whole picture is much murkier when it comes to carbohydrates. All the sugars, starch (potatoes, apples), cellulose (the stringy bits in vegetables like celery), gum, pectin (the gummy component of fruit that makes jam set), and many other compounds are members of the carbohydrate family. Essentially, they are

LIVING LONGER

It has become clear that for people with very high levels of serum cholesterol, reducing the total amount of fat they eat in their diet, particularly the amount of saturated fat, helps lower their cholesterol level, and that does reduce their risk of a heart attack. In short, they live longer.

This evidence comes simply from long-term studies of groups of high-risk people who either did or did not change their dietary habits.

Most of us have much lower levels of serum cholesterol, which nonetheless constitute a significant risk factor for heart disease. What is not yet established is whether we too can derive the same benefit from a fairly drastic change in diet, namely cutting down on fats generally and substituting saturated fats with polyunsaturated fats.

My own view is that we should alter our diets because there are many other benefits from a reduction in fats, not least being that you'll cut many calories from your diet because fats are the most caloric foods. While eating unsaturated fats may not be a complete panacea (they contain just the same amount of calories as saturated fats), for the time being, at least, they are certainly healthier. Fish oils are the healthiest because the oil seems to protect against heart disease, and I recommend that you eat oily fish twice a week.

WHY FIBER IS HEALTHY

In the developing world, where unrefined plant material, in the form of roots and wholegrains, makes up the majority of the diet, conditions such as diverticular disease, hemorrhoids, appendicitis, and bowel cancer are virtually unknown.

Much of what we regard as roughage is actually soluble, and forms a sticky, viscous gel in the gut, rather like oatmeal. It acts as a cleansing agent – like a sponge – absorbing toxic and potentially hazardous compounds as it passes through.

It is now well established that a regular diet rich in soluble fiber can also reduce the level of low-density lipoproteins in the bloodstream (see p. 60). Quite apart from potentially reducing the risk of coronary artery disease, a reduction in circulating cholesterol may also reduce the risk of gallstones (which are formed from crystals of cholesterol).

Another consequence of eating a reasonable amount of fiber is that it helps food pass through the gut more quickly. Thus any toxins or potential carcinogens have less time to act on the lining of the gut. Colon cancer is a disease of affluent countries that shows a significant correlation with diet, both with high levels of fat and low levels of dietary fiber. Although we can't yet with absolute certainty isolate a particular culprit, it is a further argument for prudent adjustment of both.

all made from simple sugar units such as glucose, or its near relatives, and they all, ultimately, come from the interaction of the sun with plants, as a result of photosynthesis. While the sugars with small molecules such as fructose (fruit sugar) and lactose (milk sugar) are water-soluble, the larger ones – the polysaccharides like starch and cellulose – are insoluble. Apart from two important secondary sources of sugar – honey and breast milk – we should obtain all our carbohydrate from fruits and vegetables – in other words from plant material.

Cellulose Plants have cellulose as we have skeletons – to provide them with a framework of support. They use large-moleculed starch to store energy and they use the small-moleculed soluble sugars to transport energy and release it. The human body can digest sugar and, if it's cooked or fermented, can digest starch, but the body cannot break down cellulose. Cellulose remains in the gut as "fiber" or bulk.

Since the mid-nineteenth century we have tended to regard cellulose and all the other indigestible parts of plants as inconveniences to be avoided. Great store was put on refined and more easily digestible extracts of plants, such as white flour, white rice, and peeled potatoes. By refining plant material, we isolate the energy sources and concentrate them. The most concentrated and refined source of carbohydrate energy is, of course, sugar. Until the 1970s, this urge to refine foods was thought to be beneficial, but now we know better. By separating the essential energy of plants from all the rest, we not only lose some of the nutritional components – valuable protein, minerals, vitamins, and oils – but we also lose the fiber.

Fiber The medical significance of fiber has been known for more than 25 years but it became prominent with Audrey Eyton's F-Plan diet, one of the most successful diets in recent times. Fiber is now recognized to have several valuable properties. The most obvious is the bulk effect. Fiber bulks up the contents of our intestines and so makes our stools less dense and more soft. This can lead to a bloated feeling when you first increase the amount of fiber in your diet, but there are many positive benefits that outweigh this temporary discomfort. In addition to the health benefits (see column, left), there is one more extremely important bonus that comes from eating food in a more natural and bulkier form: the goodness within it is surrendered more gradually. This means that the rate at which your blood glucose level rises after a meal is slower and this affects your mood, so that by eating wholefoods you get fewer troughs of low blood sugar when cravings can arise.

CARBOHYDRATES AND MOODS

Most of us appreciate the odd cookie or danish but, whereas that may satisfy the appetite, carbohydrate cravers (see p. 75) may continue to eat until they have consumed snacks with the caloric value of a large meal. These snacks are over and above the body's energy needs and, because they invariably consist of refined carbohydrates such as sugar, they are likely to be converted into fat.

For most people, eating a sugar-rich snack when they're hungry triggers the release of insulin in an attempt to stabilize the blood-sugar level. A couple of hours after a sugary snack, the insulin has successfully mopped up most of the glucose circulating in the blood, which can leave you suddenly very short of energy, a condition known as rebound hypoglycemia. In sharp contrast, most carbohydrate cravers feel better and refreshed, and therefore end up eating more carbohydrates simply for the good feeling this induces. Many carbohydrate cravers show a marked susceptibility to depression. Not surprisingly, cravers hardly ever eat because of hunger, but usually because of fatigue, anxiety, or tension; carbohydrates make them feel calmer and more clear-headed.

The immediate response to a carbohydrate binge is the release of large amounts of insulin into the bloodstream. An indirect consequence of this is that an increased amount of the amino acid tryptophan gets into the brain, where it is converted into serotonin, one of the brain's messenger molecules. Serotonin appears to act on the "satiety center," which controls appetite for carbohydrates. In practice, the sugar from a cookie quickly reaches the bloodstream; insulin is released, more tryptophan gets into the brain and is synthesized into serotonin, and the appetite is satisfied. It is possible that with a carbohydrate craver, this feedback system doesn't work as quickly to turn off the craving. Or it may simply be that cravers eat to control their mood rather than because they are hungry.

HIGH-SUGAR DIET

Since the advent of refined sugar our bodies have come to rely much more on the regulating role of insulin.

Among the diseases of affluence, adult-onset diabetes is yet another that shows a striking association with the Western diet. The incidence of diabetes in undeveloped countries is very low but it rises markedly with urbanization and the consumption of more refined foods. It may be that the sheer concentration of glucose rapidly absorbed into the bloodstream and assaulting the beta cells of the pancreas (where insulin is synthesized and released) is a direct cause of the disease.

We in the Western world seem to have developed a tolerance to much higher concentrations of blood glucose than the levels to which our bodies have been accustomed through evolution. When levels begin to drop, we may have cravings for sweet foods or anything that serves the same purpose (for example, a liquid lunch).

The trouble with getting glucose in such a way is that afterward your blood sugar level plummets and you become irritable, impatient, and short-tempered. Your concentration goes and so does your ability to make decisions.

You can avoid this state of affairs if you eat carbohydrate every two hours, as I suggest in my eating plan, to keep your blood sugar levels even.

THE HEART-HEALTHY DIET

Our choice of food, the way we choose to cook it, and especially the amount we eat do indeed affect our health. The wrong eating pattern over a period of time combined with other bad habits, such as smoking, excessive drinking and insufficient exercise, can lead to disease and early death. The most striking correlation between what we eat and illness is between saturated fat (found almost entirely in meat and dairy products) and coronary artery disease. The connection is made through that infamous and much maligned intermediate mentioned earlier, cholesterol.

Cholesterol lies at the center of the great diet-disease debate. Speaking in general terms, the more saturated fat you eat, the more cholesterol will be found in your bloodstream, and the higher your (serum) cholesterol level, the greater the risk of an early death from coronary artery disease. However, serum cholesterol is only one of several risk factors in coronary artery disease, and our cholesterol level is mainly determined by cholesterol manufactured inside the body.

In coronary artery disease, the buildup of fat (atheroma) in the lining of the coronary arteries gradually narrows them and consequently the blood supply to the muscles of the heart is reduced. A heart attack happens when one of the major coronary arteries is completely blocked by a blood clot (thrombus) forming in a matter of hours around a particularly prominent fatty deposit on the lining of the artery wall. Some people experience severe chest pains (angina) in the weeks preceding a heart attack; others get no early warning.

The important point is this: there is a wealth of data, accumulated over decades, to support these findings – namely that the level of cholesterol in the bloodstream is our best indicator of the risk of coronary artery disease. This is not the same thing as saying that cholesterol causes heart attacks. Few scientists are satisfied that cause and effect has been proven. Even if it is entirely free of blame, however, as an indicator, high levels of cholesterol tell us to cut down on our dietary intake of fats – particularly saturated fats – because this will reduce our risk of heart disease. This is the simple and vital take-home message.

Watch your alcohol
It is now well known that habits such as smoking and regularly drinking too much alcohol, can contribute to or cause certain illnesses.

STAYING SLIM AND HEALTHY

By and large being slim is usually much healthier than being obese. Or to look at it another way, the good news is that if you eat healthily, you're almost certain to be slim. Most of us can find the will-power to lose a bit of weight, it's keeping it off that really tests us. However, it isn't that hard if you acquire some healthy eating habits, such as getting most of your calories from unrefined carbohydrate (whole-wheat bread, pasta, rice, cereals, and legumes), and eating more fruit and vegetables. This also deals with food cravings – you'll find that if you eat plenty of unprocessed carbohydrate, you don't need to resort to bingeing.

DECISION TIME

There is little point in giving you a long list of "don'ts" and, anyway, I don't believe I should proscribe any foods. The only way to lose weight and stay slim for the rest of your life is to control your intake of energy-rich foods, namely fats and sugars. If you adopt my guidelines, I know you'll find the food both appetizing and filling and, even more important, you'll find it's much easier than you imagined to take control of your eating pattern.

Look at your present eating habits and decide where you can make appropriate substitutions. Remember though, even as you eat more and more fresh fruit and vegetables as your primary source of sugar, whenever you do eat a sugary snack you are adding calories with little or no nutritional value.

CUTTING OUT SUGAR

The food industry has slowly responded to the growing demand for low-sugar or sugar-free products. Many canned fruits are now available in fruit juice, still rich in natural sugar but a great improvement on syrup. Sugar-free baked beans are also now widely available and make an excellent convenience food. It's up to you to check what exactly is in what you are buying. Look at the labels and if it's not clear, ask the store manager. It's only by customers bringing the issue to the retailers' attention that they will increase their range of low-sugar or sugar-free products.

I know that cutting down on sugar may be the hardest change for you to make. Please persevere! Sugar is such a potent food that the body does acquire a sugar habit and it will take time to kick it.

Healthy snacks Don't forget that unprocessed carbohydrates, such as whole-wheat bread and pasta, rice, potatoes (with their skins), and oatmeal, are the dieter's best friends because they curb craving, smooth out blood-sugar levels, and can make you feel satisfied for four or more hours. Snack on this kind of carbohydrate between meals, and keep ample supplies in the refrigerator. You've got to eat about 4oz (100g) of carbohydrate to stave off cravings – that's the equivalent of two slices of whole-wheat bread.

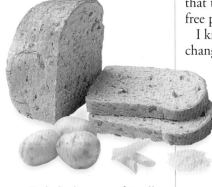

Carbohydrates are friendly
Change your diet to include more unrefined carbohydrates, such as pasta, bread, and potatoes in your daily diet to curb cravings and bingeing.

NUTRITIONAL GUIDELINES

To eat a well-balanced and healthy diet you need to eat the right types and proportions of foods, with the emphasis on fruit and vegetables and complex carbohydrates like bread and rice. Based on the latest scientific research, the Food and Drug Administration recommends the following daily quantities for those not on a diet; all items in italic represent one measure.

6–14 measures of bread, other cereals, and potatoes

2–3 tbsp breakfast cereal
or muesli
1 slice bread/toast
3 crackers/crispbreads

2 heaping tbsp rice
3 heaping tbsp pasta
2 egg-sized boiled
potatoes

5 or more measures of fruit and vegetables

medium-sized fresh fruit
a medium portion of
vegetables or salad

6 tbsp stewed/canned fruit
1 small glass of fruit juice

2–3 measures of milk and dairy foods

1 medium glass of milk
1 small container of yogurt
1 large portion of
cottage cheese

1 large portion of
fromage frais
1 matchbox-sized piece
of cheese

2–4 measures of meat, fish, and alternatives

2 medium slices of beef,
pork, ham, lamb, liver,
chicken, or fish
2 eggs

5 tbsp baked beans
4 tbsp cooked lentils
2 tbsp nuts or peanut
butter

1–5 measures of the following foods that contain fat

1 tsp butter or margarine
1 tsp oil

2 tsp low-fat spread

Avoid, but no more than 2 measures of the following foods that contain fat

1 packet potato chips   *1 tbsp cream*   *1 tbsp mayonnaise*

Avoid, but no more than 2 measures of the following foods that contain sugar

3 tsp sugar
1 heaping tsp jam/honey
2 cookies

1 small chocolate bar
1 small bag of candy
half a slice of cake

FLUID

About 55–65 percent of the human body is made up of water, but this is constantly being lost through urine and feces, perspiration, and physical exertion.

The loss is even greater in hot temperatures. To help the body function properly, this fluid has to be replaced. Some water comes from foods, especially fruit and vegetables, but it's also essential to drink an adequate amount. Aim to drink 6–8 large glasses of fluid a day. Although any fluid is better than no fluid, pure water is best, followed by fruit juices and low-fat milk. Drinks that contain caffeine, such as tea, coffee, and some cola drinks, are not as good for maintaining water balance since they make us excrete more urine.

ALCOHOL RECOMMENDATIONS

Women should drink no more than 2–3 units of alcohol per day, and men no more than 3–4 units. Remember, alcohol is high in calories, so if you're trying to lose weight it's better not to drink any at all.

One unit is:
- *half a pint of ordinary-strength beer or lager*
- *1 small glass of wine*
- *1 ounce measure of hard liquor*

MAKING THE CHANGE TO HEALTHIER EATING

The benefits of a healthy lifestyle based on regular exercise and a good diet will quickly become apparent and, like me, you'll probably wonder how you ever managed to get by previously. You will feel better and find you have more energy. But switching to a healthy lifestyle will put you in the vanguard of the nation's health movement and by becoming a forward thinker you will have to put up with other more backward thinkers all around you. In practice, this means that you have to rely more on yourself and less on others for maintaining your healthy diet.

All of you will probably have nagging doubts about how feasible the changes are. How much hardship is involved? Will the inconvenience be too much for you? Will the restrictions be demoralizing? Well, there have been a number of studies looking at how easily people cope with changing to healthy eating. One that I found particularly interesting involved a group of nearly 500 dieticians and their families who, instead of changing gradually, agreed to make the switch overnight.

Of course, some found it easier than others to make the changes. Many thought that they could adjust overnight to the new eating pattern that would last for the rest of their lives. Many commented on the need to eat larger meals more frequently because the food they were now eating was not as rich in calories as their previous diet. This happens when you substitute unprocessed carbo-hydrates such as whole grains, pasta, rice, and legumes for rich fatty foods and refined sugary foods.

It's good news for anybody who is overweight because eating the right foods automatically reduces your calorie intake – even if you feel you are eating more volume overall. What's more, although there are fewer calories, there are more nutrients, so you win both ways!

Jogging
If you exercise regularly, you can eat well and still keep slim. Enjoy exercising at home to music. It will bring a healthy glow to your face too.

PREPARATION, EFFORT, AND TIME

Every change works best if you're prepared – I found that out when I made a TV series on how to give up smoking. So I feel I must warn you about your hardest job. Substituting unprocessed starchy food for rich, fatty foods is the single most important aspect of the transition to healthier eating and, as the dieticians' study revealed, this is the switch that also takes the most effort.

After all, the message to cut down on sugar, in the name of less dental decay, has only been really successful in the last few years. Given that saturated fat has been exposed as a "villain" comparatively recently and the mistaken victim, starch, has been allowed a slow rehabilitation, it's going to take a little time for that message to build in strength and be acted on.

Quite apart from the mental adjustment needed when planning menus along the new guidelines, the dieticians mentioned earlier found that they had to plan ahead when shopping and stockpile healthy snacks whenever they came across them because these foods are not stocked by all supermarkets. To be forewarned is to be forearmed!

I suggest that you set yourself a timetable for the transition. Don't try to do everything at once – start by reducing your intake of red meat for example, and the following week, perhaps, change to low-fat milk. If you intend to convert your family with you, you will have to take care to make such changes gradually.

Fresh fruit
All fruits are good natural sources of energy, vitamins, minerals, and fiber. Eat plenty during the day as snacks, or after your main meals for dessert.

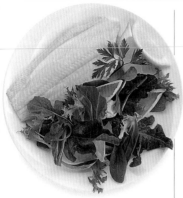

Eat more fish
All fish, but in particular oily fish, are good sources of vitamins, minerals and unsaturated fats. They also provide a delicious and healthy alternative to fatty red meat.

YOUR NEW ACTION PLAN FOR EATING

In addition to eating well and wisely, you now need to change the way you choose and prepare your food. None of these changes will be news to you but they will help you to adjust the ratio of fat to starch in your diet.

Fats
• Start by cutting down on fatty meals: broil rather than fry food; eat more boiled or baked potatoes and avoid fried or roast potatoes.
• Use skim or low-fat milk instead of whole milk.
• Make sure that the oil you use is unsaturated (for example, sunflower, corn, olive, or canola oil) and not just labeled "vegetable oil," since it may be a blend containing saturated oil.
• Use an unsaturated margarine and spread it thinly over your whole-wheat bread.

Meat
• Stop cooking "meat and two vegetables" meals. Start cooking more vegetables with less meat.
• Eat more white meat and fish or leaner cuts of the red meats. Be careful: even "lean" cuts of beef, pork, and lamb contain small percentages of fat. Sausages, ground beef, burgers, and pâtés are very high in fat, much of it saturated.
• Liver, kidneys, and organ meat in general tend to be far less fatty than red meat, so eat more of these.
• When you cook chicken or other fowl, don't eat the skin, which is rich in fat.
• Stir-fries are an excellent way to make a tasty meal using less meat and less fat. You need only a little oil and seasoning in a hot wok. Stir-frying is also more economical on heat and makes clearing up simpler.

Salt
• Try to phase out the practice of adding extra salt to your food over a few weeks. If you really must have salt, use much less and use it only while cooking.
• Never leave chopped vegetables in salted water and throw away salted vegetable water.

• Beans, legumes, and lentils will cook more quickly and without hardening if you cut out salt.

• If you cook pasta in salted water, rinse it with boiling water before serving.

• If food tastes flat without salt to begin with, be patient. Give your palate time to reset at a new level. Once you and your family have adjusted to low-salt or salt-free cooking, you'll wonder what all the fuss was about. Experiment – there are many ways to enhance and supplement the natural flavors of food without resorting to salt. Herbs and spices are particularly good and there are so many to choose from. Try using black pepper, paprika, nutmeg, cumin, or a mixture of spices.

• Of course, there are low-sodium salts (based on potassium instead of sodium) that can help some people but I hesitate to recommend them for nonmedical diets since it seems to me to be an admission of defeat.

• Banishing the salt cellar from the house is not the end of the matter. Most of the salt we eat is already included in food produce: bacon and smoked fish and meats are quite high in salt; pickles, sauces, canned soups and most of the savory snack foods such as nuts, potato chips and nibbles are all quite heavily salted. So cut down on these processed foods.

• Be careful: other sources of salt are less obvious. Canned fish and vegetables, breakfast cereals, and some of the hard cheeses can also contain appreciable quantities of salt.

• Remember, we are not trying to remove all salt from the diet – a little salt is an absolute physiological necessity – especially in hot climates.

Sugar

• Sugar (sucrose) only contains calories. It has no nutritional value whatsoever. White and brown sugar should be avoided completely.

• However, even if you throw away your sugar bowl, there are other sources of sugar to watch out for. Sugar alone, or when added to processed food, comes in many forms other than that labeled "sugar" or "sucrose." These other kinds, which are all just as much of a problem, include glucose, maltose, fructose, any syrup (for example, dextrose, glucose), and any type of sugar – whether or not it is called unrefined – for example, cane sugar, molasses, muscovado, and demerara.

WHERE'S THE HIDDEN SUGAR?

All types of sugars permeate a huge proportion of the food industry's products because their ability to enhance flavors is highly valued. It's important that you become aware of quite how extensively sugar is used even in savory products such as ketchup and bread.

• *About 60 percent of the hundreds of millions of tons of sugar consumed in the US each year is eaten in the form of processed foods. Of course, chocolate and all candies account for a large part of that consumption; a large proportion of the rest comes from cookies, sweet pastries, cakes, jams and other spreads, pickles, chutneys, and sauces.*

• *Most bottled drinks have a high sugar content, as do most ice creams and dessert dishes.*

• *Unless plain yogurt is specifically labeled "very low calorie" it is very likely to have added sugar.*

• *Most of the popular processed breakfast cereals have a surprisingly high sugar content. A few make a point of being sugar-free – look for them.*

• *Because sugar is such an excellent preservative, many canned foods are packaged in syrup, so beware! Many fruits are now available in natural fruit juice.*

KEEPING IT GOING

The weakness in many diets is that they fail to help you maintain your desired weight once you have reached it. Most of us have at some time or other dieted sufficiently strictly to get down to the weight we were aiming for, but nearly everyone will confess that they didn't stay at their ideal weight for long. This is because most diets do not train you to eat in a way that can be sustained happily for the long term. My eating plan is different: while the seven-day diet is fairly rigid, the essential aspects of it still provide an excellent way to continue to eat for the rest of your life. You have already learned about the bonuses of eating my way; you do not feel hungry, you do not get cravings, you do not binge, so, in the long run, you will not put the weight back on. The principles of the seven-day eating plan are so sound that they can be applied to general everyday living, not just to keep you trim but also to keep you in good health.

YOUR FAVORITE FOODS

One of the reasons why people find it difficult to stick to healthy eating is that they believe they have to abandon all their favorite foods for the rest of their lives; this is not true with my eating plan. It is a lifestyle not a life sentence, and it is an eating plan not a diet. I have a rule that I call the 80/20 rule, passed on to me by an American colleague who is an expert in long-term healthy eating:

If you eat the right food for 80 percent of the time, it hardly matters what you eat for the other 20 percent.

So there is no need to pine for treat foods – you can have them sometimes – and there is no need to deprive yourself to the point where you are overcome by cravings and so binge on your treat foods. Remember the 80/20 rule and it will help you keep a balanced perspective on what you eat and the way that you eat it.

CHANGING YOUR EATING HABITS

Changing our eating habits can be an inconvenience that cuts right through our daily lives and it is one major reason why so many people find ordinary dieting hard work. But with this eating plan it won't be hard work, it will be less painful than you ever imagined. This is a guide to healthy eating for everyone; young and old, singles and families, and it is never too late to start. You will feel and see the benefits immediately.

I have drawn up easy eating guidelines for you to follow, if you want to, for the rest of your life. The decision is yours and yours alone. However, if you are on a special diet for medical reasons, for example, if you have diabetes, hypertension, a food allergy, or you are receiving any medication, it would be wise to consult your doctor before starting my plan. But, unless this is the case, there's no need to worry because my guidelines are the culmination of years of my interpretation on your behalf of research, discussions, committees, and reports from the experts. What's more, my guidelines are also shaped by common sense because, having been a failed dieter all my life, I know the pitfalls. I have devised an eating plan based on good science and how the body works, but which is nonetheless easy to follow.

MAKING IT WORK FOR THE LONG TERM

You've started to lose weight on the first part of the eating plan (and can continue to trim your body by simply repeating the first seven days) but if you're anything like me, you must be wondering how you're going to keep it off. I honestly don't think I'm exaggerating when I say it isn't going to be difficult – at least not as difficult as you may think and certainly not as difficult as it may have been before. I'll even go so far as to say that you won't have to stay on a totally regimented eating plan either. Sounds far-fetched? Let me explain.

The mainstay of my eating plan is to eat a little *often and regularly*. There are at least two pay-offs from this: first, if you eat every two hours you're hardly ever hungry; second, as eating activates the body's metabolism, you burn more calories every day than you do when you eat sparingly and infrequently, and you use a tremendous amount more calories than you would if you tried to lose weight by going on a crash diet, starvation diet, or microdiet. So with my eating plan, you can eat great food, cook delicious recipes, look good and feel good, and still lose weight – and it will stay off!

DISPELLING A FEW MYTHS ABOUT FOOD

All of us have heard certain ideas about food that we accept as the truth but they are not necessarily correct. The following may help you think again:

- *No food in itself is slimming.*

- *Water retention is thought to be at the root of weight gain for some people. Unfortunately, for most of us, the rule of thumb is that it never is.*

- *It is thought that when dieting, initial weight loss is mainly due to water loss. It is if you starve yourself, but it isn't with my eating plan.*

CHANGING A FEW BAD HABITS

You're going to have to change a few habits, of course, but as I describe them you'll know in your heart of hearts that this is not really difficult. Many years ago I tried changing my family's diet (husband and four sons) and it worked almost without them noticing. I had just returned from making a TV program in California about preventing heart disease and was bursting with enthusiasm for a new heart-healthy diet. At breakfast I announced the new regime, saying that at the end of a fortnight's trial we would vote on it. When the two weeks were up I offered, "Well, how's the skim milk going down, the lack of butter, the whole-wheat bread...?" The responses came, "What bread?" "Isn't the milk the same?" "Didn't miss butter." Healthy eating had become the norm, painlessly, for the whole family.

This experience with my own family made me realize that healthy eating habits, which some people dread, are much easier to incorporate into your life than you think. If you're worried about the lack of salt, there's no need for your food to be less tasty if you take advantage of the natural sodium that is found in herbs and spices. All you have to do is release that sodium by "sweating" some finely chopped herbs, onions, and crushed garlic in a skillet with a tiny amount of oil and then adding the mixture to your cooking.

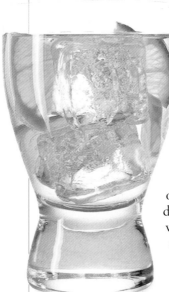

Many people manage without sugar in tea and coffee, so why don't you give it up altogether? In my own case, I gave up sugar many years ago when I first became pregnant. I calculated that I'd eat and drink a massive amount of sugar in nine months and so I decided that I, and my baby, could well do without it. You could use artificial sweeteners instead if you like them, or why not just phase out your taste for sugar gradually by taking a little less each time.

Water
Keep a pitcher of cool water in the refrigerator and drink plenty throughout the day. Try it with ice and lemon.

EATING CARBOHYDRATES TO STAY SLIM

My eating plan concentrates on carbohydrates (starch) – not empty refined starch like white bread, cakes, candy, and so on, but unrefined starches: fruit and vegetables, whole grains, beans, peas, and legumes; brown rice and, particularly, potatoes. With my eating plan you can even have a carbohydrate blow-out and eat 1lb (0.5kg) of potatoes if you want to.

This is for very good reasons: it's following good nutritional theory to make carbohydrates the linchpin of any eating plan because they are bulky and make you feel full; they improve the function of the bowels (see p. 62); they flatten off sudden peaks of high blood sugar that inevitably end in low blood sugar levels and a craving for sugar. The truth is that the only way to treat a carbohydrate craving is to eat carbohydrate – but you should eat unrefined starch, not a chocolate bar.

CARBOHYDRATE CRAVINGS

People who crave chocolate and sweet things typically snack in the late afternoon and early evening. My eating plan tries to anticipate this craving by scheduling an unprocessed starch meal around late afternoon when your blood glucose level may be dropping. This slow-release form of carbohydrate should help to turn off the craving without having to resort to sugary snacks (which may exacerbate it). Give your body a little time to adjust and be gentle with yourself. Instead of a chocolate bar eat a small potato in its skin, a cupful of rice, or a plate of dahl. You'll have to be mature enough to forego the instant gratification that chocolate and sweet things can give, but this really does work.

Starchy carbohydrates are the dieter's best friend because they make you feel good. Proteins don't, which is why it's very difficult to stick to a high-protein diet. If you base your eating on carbohydrates, as my eating plan suggests, you reduce the chances of getting depressed, giving in to a craving, or even giving up the whole thing.

You've got to get the right kind of carbohydrates into your diet because they make controlled eating easier; in fact, they give you control. The best way to stay slim is to eat carbohydrates every two hours because, unlike most diets, it works *with* your body instead of *against* it.

COPING WITH DIFFICULT MEALTIMES

Ah, eating sensibly is all very well, you're saying, but life isn't always that easy. What about the business lunch? What about only having time for a snack or eating on the run? Do I resort to old habits? You needn't. Here's how.

THE BUSINESS LUNCH

The key to the successful business lunch is to see it as a treat. You can have the most delicious food, which is also healthy and low in calories:

Aperitif
Have a large glass of mineral water, which will start to fill you up so that you will eat less.

Appetizer Choose one of the following:
• Vegetable soup
• Smoked salmon
• Gravadlax
• Half an Ogen melon or other fruits
• A gorgeous salad (ask for the dressing on the side so that you can add only what you want)
• Fresh shrimp (without mayonnaise or butter)
• Eat the bread roll if it's whole-wheat, but no butter

Main course Choose one of the following:
• Steamed or grilled fish but choose the nicest (for example, monkfish, turbot, halibut, and swordfish)
• Grilled chicken breast (no skin)
• A vegetarian dish
• At least four vegetables (exclude potatoes this time); they help satisfy you so eat them FIRST
• Dishes without creamy sauces
• Any amount of salad

Dessert
• Fresh fruit is the best option but choose the most appetizing and exotic, for example, mango, papaya, passion fruit, guavas, raspberries, and strawberries out of season. Or you could simply opt for a fresh fruit salad.
• Avoid cheese and cookies – they are high in calories

Wine
One glass of white, red, or rosé

Water
Drink a glass of water for every glass of wine, plus an extra glass of water

Coffee
Drink it black, without cream or sugar

Liqueurs
Pass on the port, brandy, and sweet liqueurs

FOOD ON THE RUN

• Keep a piece of fruit (an apple or banana) and/or a small piece of Dutch or Swiss cheese handy
• Buy ½lb (0.25kg) of your favorite fruit or a low-calorie cereal bar and eat them on the run
• Drink 1½ cups (0.25 liter) of skim or low-fat, but not whole milk
• Have a bowl of verylow-fat, flavored yogurt and a plain whole-wheat roll
• Have a portion of any salad, but leave as much of the dressing as you can
• Avoid salads with mayonnaise dressings if possible
• Don't eat potato chips: they are high in fat and salt
• Don't be tempted by chocolate bars or cookies

Sandwiches Make your own sandwiches or ask the deli to make them using:
• Whole-wheat or granary bread or rolls
• No butter or margarine
• No dressing of any kind
• Lots of black pepper (if liked)

Takeout food
• Drop into a Greek takeout and grab a pitta with a little lean meat, chicken, or houmous, and lots of salad
• If you're having an Indian meal, just ask for a dish of dahl or vegetables and a chappati or boiled rice
• When going for a Chinese takeout, ask for a dish of mixed vegetables and plenty of boiled rice
• Avoid fried takeout foods such as egg rolls and fish and french fries entirely

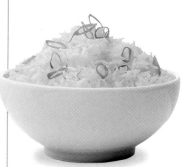

Fast but healthy food
A bowl of rice served with stir-fried vegetables, chicken, fish, or even on its own, is nutritious, filling, and is also easy to make.

77

TIPS ON HOW
TO CHEAT YOUR
APPETITE

If you feel hungry, you may be tempted to eat too much or the wrong type of food. Follow these tips to keep hunger at bay:

- *Eat before you get really hungry so that you're more likely to be satisfied with small portions of food.*

- *Always serve your food on a small plate so that you're not tempted to give yourself too much food.*

- *Eat the healthier parts of the meal first, such as the vegetables, salad, or fruit, and eat the meat last.*

- *Eat very slowly to allow the carbohydrates to act and turn off your appetite.*

- *If you want to nibble, eat rice, legumes, or cold potatoes.*

- *Drink water all through the day and especially at mealtimes; hunger pains are often brought on by thirst.*

- *Eat filling foods such as oats, kidney beans, and beets, and anything else that contains soluble fiber.*

- *Learn to recognize when you are comfortably full, instead of eating to bursting point.*

- *Take a 20-minute break after your main course to find out if you are really still hungry.*

SWEET CRAVINGS

You may now be feeling very hungry and having cravings for your favorite sweets or creamy foods. Don't despair, this is a normal stage in any diet and there are ways around these problems. Try out my tips (see column, left) to help beat those hunger pangs. You could also make my alternative treat sweets (below) that do not contain sugar but taste just as good.

SWEET TREATS

For the incorrigible sweet tooth, here are a couple of recipes for sweet treats that you can eat once or twice a week instead of candy, chocolate, and ice cream. One of these could even be eaten during the seven-day diet if you are *in extremis*!

Apricot and Orange Balls (Makes about 24)
  2 cups (450g) dried apricots, chopped
  1 medium orange, peeled
    and chopped
  ⅔ cup (65g) grated coconut
  ½ cup (65g) ground nuts

1 Mix all the ingredients together; if possible, mince them in a food processor.
2 Shape the mixture into 24 small balls.
3 Chill in the refrigerator until firm.

Chewy Fruit
  1½ cups (400g) dried apricots, soaked, or fresh fruit,
    peeled and cored
  or 4 cups (800g) canned fruit in natural juices

1 Preheat the oven to its lowest setting.
2 Puree the fruit and then cook it over low heat for five minutes.
3 Cover a baking sheet with aluminum foil and put the fruit in the center. Spread it evenly across the sheet.
4 Bake the fruit in the oven for about eight hours until it becomes dry and chewy.
5 Peel it off the foil and cut into shapes. Store in the refrigerator.

SENSIBLE SHOPPING

To maintain a healthy diet, it's important to shop sensibly when you go to the supermarket. If you read food labels carefully, keep your cabinets stocked with the right basic ingredients, and buy fresh fruit and vegetables regularly, you'll have everything you need to create healthy, balanced meals.

FOOD LABELS

If you want to have more control over exactly what you eat, you are going to have to look more carefully at the products you buy off the shelf in your supermarket. Have a close look at the packages in your freezer and the cans in your cabinets.

Information on food labels is usually given in the same way and is governed in the US by the Center for Food Safety and Applied Nutrition (CFSAN). The regulations cover all the information on the label, including nutritional details, food storage guidelines, and ingredients (including additives).

Nutrition labeling is required on nearly all packaged foods in the United States. Nutritional information must be presented in a specific way. The grams of fat, protein, and total carbohydrate, and milligrams of cholesterol and sodium, per serving are always listed, as well as the calories (kcal). The carboydrate is usually broken down into grams of fiber and grams of sugars, and the fat may be divided into saturated and unsaturated. Manufacturers are encouraged to provide this additional information to help the consumer make suitable choices. Other nutrients can be included voluntarily but if a claim is made about them the amounts must be specified as a percentage of the daily recommended value; vitamins and minerals will only be included if they are present in significant amounts.

Read all food and beverage labels carefully: a fruit juice labeled "no added sugar" can contain more natural sugar than a carbonated drink that admits to containing added sugar, although you will be getting some vitamins and minerals from the juice. Labels declaring high levels of vitamins and minerals need a second look too: rather than being natural ingredients, they may have been added as supplements to a processed food.

FOOD STORAGE

Since this diet suggests that you eat more legumes, fresh fruit, vegetables, and fish, your shopping and house-keeping habits will probably have to change; as you'll discover, you can't shop just once for the entire week.

• You will need to make more frequent, regular visits to the supermarket for fresh fruit and vegetables.
• Buy more fresh fish and don't keep it waiting in the refrigerator because it is most nutritious eaten on the day it is caught or bought.
• If you can, find and patronize a fresh fish store rather than accepting what's available from your local supermarket, which may be days old.
• Legumes and beans can be kept in storage jars for months but they will lose nutrients and take longer to cook, so you should buy them in relatively small quantities and replenish your supplies regularly.
• Stocks and legume dishes can take some time to cook, so prepare them in large batches when you have the time and store them in the freezer in individual-sized portions. If you have a microwave, these single servings can be quickly thawed and reheated when needed.

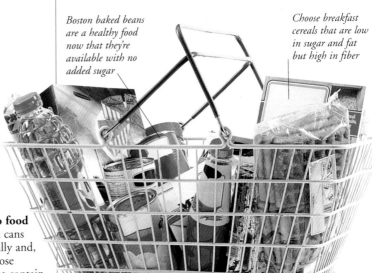

Boston baked beans are a healthy food now that they're available with no added sugar

Choose breakfast cereals that are low in sugar and fat but high in fiber

A new approach to food
Read food labels on cans and packages carefully and, where possible, choose products that do not contain added sugar or salt.

EXERCISE IN YOUR LIFE

Eating sensibly will take you 50 percent of the way to becoming trim for the rest of your life, but it isn't everything. You also need to exercise. Sadly, today, it is easy to lead a sedentary lifestyle. For many, driving to and from work, sitting in an office all day, and lying on the sofa all evening are the sum of their daily activity. If this sounds like your lifestyle, reassess it now. With my seven-day plan (see pp. 25–56), you will gradually introduce changes, so that over a week you become more physically active. Then look for ways to make sure that exercise becomes a permanent part of your lifestyle.

WHY REGULAR EXERCISE IS HEALTHY

• If you undertake regular aerobic activity, such as swimming, running, or bicycling, for at least 20 minutes at a time, your heart will become more efficient both at rest and during exercise.

• Combining regular exercise with a healthy diet will help you maintain weight loss and so prevent the conditions linked with being overweight, such as heart disease and some cancers.

• Exercising regularly will slow down the degeneration of muscles, bones, and joints as you age, and can prevent specific conditions, such as osteoporosis.

• A fit woman is less likely to develop problems when pregnant, such as excessive weight gain and varicose veins. Her recovery after childbirth is also likely to be faster if she is fit before labor.

• Exercise improves overall mental health; it improves your mood, reduces anxiety, and leaves you better able to cope with the stresses and strains of daily life.

MAINTAINING AN EXERCISE PROGRAM

Many people give up their exercise regime after a few weeks. This is often because they become bored with it or think that because they've missed one week's session, they've wrecked the program. To maintain an exercise routine you have to enjoy it and not think of it as a chore, so try to find ways to make it fun. Set yourself different challenges every week, try out new activities, and vary your routine so that it doesn't become boring. Ask a friend or your partner to join you – you're more

FINDING WAYS TO EXERCISE

Here are some simple ways to become more physically active and keep fit:

• *Try not to use an elevator or an escalator unless you have to.*

• *Walk or run, or even leap two at a time up the stairs.*

• *Walk quickly whenever you can.*

• *Always do your abdominal or tummy-flattening exercises and (for women) your Kegel exercises.*

• *Get a regular active sport going, such as tennis, squash, badminton, paddle tennis, or skiing.*

• *Take dance classes, or just go dancing socially.*

• *Invest in an exercise bike or rowing machine. Try to use it for 20–30 minutes at a time, four times a week.*

likely to go to the gym or play your exercise video if someone else is there to encourage you. If you miss one class, or you are just too tired, it doesn't mean you've failed. Think of it as a well-earned break and then start again. You can also keep fit as you go about your day-to-day activities at home: gardening and housework (especially when done vigorously) will exercise your muscles and burn calories. Make keeping fit a family event – go for long walks on the weekends, go swimming together, or just play ball with your children in the park.

ENCOURAGING CHILDREN TO EXERCISE

Most young children are always on the go, but once they're of school age, if they're driven everywhere and their leisure time mainly consists of sitting down playing computer games, it's unlikely that they're active enough. Although they will probably play some sort of sport at school, this may not be enough to keep them physically fit. This could cause problems for them in later life because, in addition to keeping fit, they need to build maximum bone mass while they're young – and this affects boys as well as girls.

Don't try to force your children to exercise in their free time if they really hate it, since this will only make them less likely to enjoy it, but you could encourage them to be more generally active. Suggest an activity on a Saturday or Sunday morning that they – or all of you – could do in the garden or the park that is more fun than watching television. Or send them on errands that will make sure they have to walk or bike.

Take them swimming from an early age and try to make this a regular activity even in adolescence. If your children are athletic types, get them involved in group sport activities: encourage them to join the local football or hockey team or suggest that they go on camping weekends with a friend.

And don't forget that you need to be a good role model for your children – if you are a nonexerciser, why should they make the effort to exercise? The best way to motivate them is to exercise regularly, stay fit, and eat well yourself.

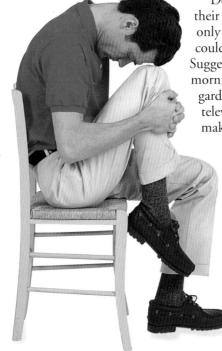

Exercise
Simple stretching exercises are beneficial to keep supple. Even when you are stuck in your office all day you can do knee-bends.

CHAPTER 5

HEALTHY EATING THROUGHOUT YOUR LIFE

Nutritional requirements soar during certain stages of your life, such as adolescence and pregnancy, so in this chapter I explain how to adapt your diet to meet your body's changing needs. There are many reasons why you might think your lifestyle is incompatible with eating in a healthy way. If you are very busy, live alone, or have a restricted budget, it's easy to forego regular meals in favor of snacks. But here you can see how a healthy, nutritious diet needn't be either expensive or time-consuming to prepare.

PUBERTY AND ADOLESCENCE

Teenagers' calorie needs are particularly high because most of them are still growing; they also spend a lot of physical and mental energy at school, in athletic activities, and in their social life. Of course, how much an individual teenager eats varies, depending on age, size, gender, and level of activity, but most eat as much as adults and sometimes much more.

If you are concerned that your teenager is eating the wrong food, then it is worthwhile trying to make unpopular meals more attractive, particularly the all-important breakfast. The easiest way is to change menus frequently. Wholegrain cereals, eggs, low-fat milk, fruit, yogurt, and low-fat cottage cheese can provide a nutritious meal but they're not to everyone's taste, and eating exactly the same food every day is boring. So it is worth providing them with more choice: for example, two cereals, several kinds of fruit, and pancakes or waffles with different toppings. You can also make breakfast interesting by offering food that is not usually served at this time, such as cheese or peanut butter sandwiches made with whole-wheat bread. Nutritious leftovers from dinner can be more interesting than cereal or eggs.

You may find it easier to interest your teenagers in the family meals if you ask them to plan the menus for a week at a time, make a chart, and post it prominently in the kitchen.

THE GROWTH SPURT

During adolescence, children reach a rate of growth second only to that of infancy. As a result of changes in the composition of their bodies, their nutritional needs change. They also differ according to their gender. The growth spurt usually begins and ends earlier in girls than in boys, so any dietary recommendations should be used only as guidelines. See the tables (pp. 86–87) for the recommended requirements for teenagers according to age, height, and weight.

Remember that parents often have little control over a teenager's eating habits. Far and away the greatest influence comes from their peers; consequently, family meals assume much less importance than they did when your children were younger. Eating becomes a social ritual that teenagers prefer to enact with their friends and they quite often like to exert greater control over their choice of foods by breaking some of the habits that are usually encouraged at home. An adolescent would be unusual if he or she were not concerned about size, shape, and image. Although boys very often want to increase their weight, many teenage girls want to decrease theirs so they cut calories. Unfortunately, many of them try to reduce their calorie intake by excluding nutritious foods such as bread, cereals, and meat, while filling up on empty high-calorie snacks and soft drinks. Probably one in four girls is trying to control her weight by some means or other, a few of which are very unhealthy; some, such as prolonged starving (anorexia) or self-inflicted vomiting (bulimia) are dangerous. If your teenager is overweight and wants to go on a reducing diet, make sure that it is a sensible one, such as the eating plan given on pages 25–56.

SNACKS AND JUNK FOOD

Surveys of teenagers show that their eating patterns change at this time so that they stop eating set meals and tend to snack. One approach, therefore, is to provide a lot of very healthy snacks and salad ingredients in the house. Breakfast and lunch are the meals most often skipped – especially by girls on diets; but patterns may also become irregular because of school activities, social demands, and part-time jobs. As a result, a teenager may take in more than what she or he needs in nutrients one day, but much less the next. Remember that it is not necessary for teenagers to meet all their food requirements every day, as long as most meals are balanced and there is an adequate intake over a period of about a week.

Besides this, there is incontrovertible evidence that adolescents can get all the nutrients they need from healthy snacks. Even some of the so-called junk foods that adults usually malign are not as low in nutrition as they may think. Nonetheless, such foods should only be eaten occasionally, rather than forming the main part of the diet.

So, armed with tables that show you the amount of food an adolescent needs from each food group, you can apply the principles of my eating plan to your teenager.

AN ADOLESCENT'S ESTIMATED AVERAGE NEEDS FOR ENERGY AND PROTEIN

	MALE		FEMALE	
Age	11–14	15–18	11–14	15–18
Weight (pounds)	98	132	98	119
(kg)	(44.5)	(60.0)	(44.5)	(54.0)
Height (in)	62	68	61	64
(cm)	(158)	(172)	(155)	(162)
Energy (calories)	2,220	2,755	1,845	2,110
Protein (oz)	1.5	1.9	1.4	1.6
(g)	42	55	41	45

DAILY FOOD GUIDE FOR ADOLESCENTS

FOOD GROUP	NUMBER OF SERVINGS	1-SERVING EQUIVALENT
Cereals and grains Wholegrain breads and cereals, brown rice, whole-wheat pasta	4 or more	1 slice of bread 1–2 cups (125–225g) cereal
Fruit and vegetables All fruits and vegetables. Be sure to include some dark-green or yellow vegetables for vitamin A and some citrus fruits or other sources of vitamin C	4 or more	1 medium fruit or vegetable ¼–½lb (125–225g)
Meat, fish, and eggs Lean meats, fish, poultry, eggs, dried peas and beans. One egg or 1 cup (125g) peas or beans or 2 tablespoons peanut butter is equal to 1oz (25g) of meat	2 or more	3–4oz (75–125g) meat, fish, or poultry
Milk and dairy products Low-fat and skim milk, plain yogurt, ice cream, cheese, and other dairy products	3 or more	2 cups (225ml) milk

A BALANCED LOW-CALORIE DIET
FOR ADOLESCENTS

MEAL	FOODS	CALORIES
Breakfast	• 1 serving fruit or juice	40
	• 6oz (175g) wholegrain ready-to eat cereal	75
	• 2 cups (225ml) low-fat milk	120
	• 1 slice whole-wheat bread	60
	• 1 tsp margarine or butter	45
	Total	**340**
Lunch	• 2oz (50g) lean meat, cheese, or fish	175
	• 2 slices whole-wheat bread	120
	• 1 tsp margarine or butter	45
	• 1 serving of vegetables or fruit	40
	• 2 cups (225g) low-fat milk	120
	Total	**500**
Dinner	• 3oz (75g) lean meat, fish, poultry, or other protein	250 40
	• 1 serving of vegetables	40
	• 1 serving of salad	
	• 1 small potato or 1 cup (125g) rice or noodles, or 1 slice whole-wheat bread	80 45
	• 1 tsp margarine or butter	40
	• 1 serving fruit	
	• 2 cups (225ml) low-fat milk	120
	Total	**615**
	Meals total	**1455**
Snacks (optional)	• 1 serving fruit	40
	• 4oz (125g) ice cream or 1 small cupcake with icing or 3 small cookies	125
	Total	**165**
	Day's total	**1620**

PREGNANT WOMEN AND BREAST-FEEDING MOTHERS

HEALTHY FOODS

You should eat a wide variety of foods from the following food groups to make sure that you're getting all the protein, minerals, and vitamins you and your baby need:

• *Milk and dairy products contain a high percentage of the protein, most of the calcium and phosphorus, and all of the vitamin D you need.*

• *Meat, fish, and poultry contain a lot of protein, B vitamins, and some iron.*

• *Vegetables, potatoes, and citrus fruits contain some protein and large quantities of vitamin C; vegetables are also an excellent source of vitamin A.*

• *Grains and cereals contain iron and B vitamins, and smaller amounts of protein, calcium, and phosphorus.*

Eating for your baby
Your body has to work very hard during pregnancy and you must eat well to maintain your health, as well as to provide the best environment for your unborn baby.

The seven-day diet given earlier in the book is so well balanced that it is perfectly safe for pregnant women and breast-feeding mothers to embark upon. In fact, it is probably better than the average diet that most women usually eat. On this healthy, well-balanced diet you will only need to make minor adjustments to accommodate any increased nutritional needs if you are pregnant.

Remember that it is essential that you do not smoke during pregnancy and most doctors recommend that you do not drink alcohol.

You should never try to lose weight when you are pregnant and, while it is normal to eat slightly more than usual during pregnancy, it is not an excuse for overeating; you should never, as the saying goes, "eat for two." In general, your energy requirements will increase by about 15 percent, which means that you will need more calories, but only 150 more calories a day during the first three months, 300 a day during the second trimester, and 400–450 during the last trimester.

Most pregnant women experience an increase in appetite. However, your digestive system is slowing down and during the last trimester the stomach takes longer to empty because the baby is pushing against it. It is important for your comfort as well as your digestion, therefore, not to overload the stomach, so my initial eating plan of five to six small meals a day is much better suited to a pregnant woman than eating fewer larger meals.

For the healthy development of your unborn baby, your diet should contain adequate protein, calcium, phosphorus, iodine, iron, and vitamins A, B, C, and D. You should also start taking folic acid supplements three months before you try to conceive and throughout pregnancy. The list (see column, left) shows which foods contain good quantities of these nutrients.

FLUIDS

During pregnancy you require a lot of liquid because your blood volume expands in order to nourish the baby, so it is a good idea to drink about 2 pints (1 liter) of low-fat milk a day and about 3 pints (1.5 liters) of other liquid. When you are breast-feeding, you will need 4 pints (2 liters) more than usual. Avoid sodas and cut back on tea and coffee – they all contain caffeine, which may not be good for the unborn baby. Do not forget that when you drink tea with a meal, the tannic acid in it can prevent your digestive system from absorbing iron from the food.

FRESH FOOD

Fresh, unprocessed foods obviously have the highest nutritional value but it may also be harmful to eat a lot of foods that contain chemical preservatives, colorings, and flavorings. Therefore, eat as much raw food as you possibly can, and buy lots of fresh fruit and vegetables. Avoid canned, frozen, and packaged convenience foods, processed meats such as sausage and pâtés, products made with refined flour, bottled sauces, and pickles, and high-calorie snacks such as chips, cookies, and candy.

FOOD SAFETY

Do not eat any food that is stale or has mold on it. Cutting off the mold does not always remove the toxins, which may have penetrated deeper into the food and which are not destroyed by cooking.

To avoid the possibility of contracting salmonella poisoning, do not eat raw eggs or products containing raw eggs, such as fresh mayonnaise and mousses, and eat eggs only if they are cooked sufficiently for the white to be firm. Do not eat unpasteurized cheeses, pre-cooked chilled foods and liver or liver pâtés. This way, you will avoid dangerous bacteria such as salmonella and listeria.

Eating well to breast-feed
It is not often realized that breast-feeding mothers need to look after themselves. They also require more calories and fluids than when they were pregnant so that they can produce ample supplies of milk for the baby.

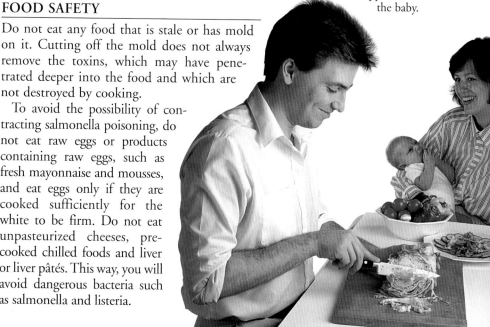

CALCIUM-RICH FOODS

It is important to eat sufficient quantities of calcium later in life. The following portions of food provide 200mg calcium:

- *1oz (25g) hard cheese*
- *2oz (50g) sardines*
- *½ cup (125g) low-fat yogurt*
- *¾ cup (175ml) low-fat milk*
- *3 cups (355g) peanuts*
- *1lb (450g) cabbage*

The richest vegetable source of calcium is broccoli. The richest source of all is dried, powdered milk, but second-best is canned salmon – as long as you eat all the bones!

FOOD FOR THE OVER-FIFTIES

Although you are getting older, it is still very important to continue to eat a varied and well-balanced diet. As a general rule, however, you will tend to be less active than when you were younger, so you will require fewer calories; also, as your metabolism slows, you will need less food. As your body ages, the digestive system slows down so you will be more comfortable if you eat smaller meals and more snacks – very much as I've suggested in the eating plan (see pp. 25–56). Your diet should consist mainly of unprocessed carbohydrates in the form of fresh fruit and vegetables, potatoes, whole-grain breads, and cereals. To help prevent the onset of osteoporosis (brittle bones), women in particular should eat lots of calcium-rich foods (see column, left).

As you get older, your food preferences may change. You'll probably find that warm foods and beverages are now easier to digest than cold ones. You will also need plenty of liquids every day, so hearty soups and stews can provide delicious ways to fulfill most of your nutritional requirements.

YOUR EATING HABITS

With increasing age, we tend to become absent-minded and it is easy to neglect the diet. If you find this is your problem, you must devise ways to overcome it. So, for example, impose set mealtimes for yourself and plan all your meals and snacks ahead one day at a time. Write down a plan first thing in the morning after breakfast and put it in a prominent place. Another way to prompt yourself to eat regularly is to have at least one healthy snack a day with a friend, a neighbor, or a member of the family, or possibly while watching your favorite television program or while you listen to the radio.

Even if you have never eaten a healthy diet before, it is never too late to start. Set yourself realistic goals and make changes to your diet very gradually, making only one change (such as changing from whole milk to low-fat milk) per week. Be sure to tell your family and friends about the changes that you are making to your diet and ask them to support you.

DIETING ON A BUDGET

It's a common myth that in order to eat well you have to spend a lot of money. This is simply not true. In fact, a healthy diet based around balanced, home-cooked meals and plenty of fruit and vegetables is much cheaper than a diet of potato chips, candy, and convenience foods.

Most of us have to survive on a limited budget at some point in our lives. If money is tight, here are some ideas to help make your food budget stretch further.

• down and make a list of everything you need before you go to the supermarket.

• Have a snack before you set out. If you feel hungry while you are shopping, you might buy more than you need.

• Make the most of foods that are in season.

• Don't buy prepared meals.

• Keep and use discount coupons – every little bit helps.

• Buy fruit and vegetables from your local market. Try shopping there late on Saturday afternoons when the merchants sell produce at reduced prices.

Some foods are much better value than others. The following table may help you to make some prudent decisions – both for your pocket and for your health!

VALUE-FOR-MONEY FOODS

FOODS	MORE NUTRITION FOR YOUR MONEY	LESS NUTRITION FOR YOUR MONEY
Meat	Poultry: chicken, turkey	Beef, lamb
	Game: pheasant, pigeon, partridge, rabbit, venison	Manufactured pork and game pies
	Liver and other organ meats	Processed meats
	Homemade burgers and meat products from lean minced steak or other meat	Manufactured burgers, meat pâtés, spreads, and speciality sausages
	Low-fat sausages	Standard sausages

VALUE-FOR-MONEY FOODS (CONTINUED)

Food	More nutrition for your money	Less nutrition for your money
Fish	Plain frozen fish (no additives)	Fish frozen with polyphosphates or in sauces
	Homemade fish fingers and fishcakes	Packaged fish fingers and other fish in batter
	Fresh fish, canned tuna, sardines, and mackerel	Canned fish in sauces and canned shellfish
Bread and cereals	Breads: whole-wheat, wheatgerm, granary, mixed grain, sprouted seed, pumpernickel, and rye	White bread and rolls
		Croissants and other sweetened breads
	Sugar-free breakfast cereals	Breakfast cereals containing sugar, salt, and food coloring
	Oatmeal	Instant hot cereals
Fats	Soft vegetable margarines high in polyunsaturates	Hard and soft margarines low in polyunsaturates, dairy spreads, low-fat spreads
	Unsalted butter	Salted butter
	Polyunsaturated vegetable oils, e.g., sunflower, safflower, corn	Drippings, lard, suet, blended cooking oils
	Homemade salad dressings, e.g., oil and vinegar dressing	Bottled or other commercial salad dressings

FOOD	MORE NUTRITION FOR YOUR MONEY	LESS NUTRITION FOR YOUR MONEY
Vegetables	Fresh fruit and vegetables in season	Bruised and overripe fruit and vegetables
	Fruit canned in its own juice or water	Fruit canned in syrup
	Vegetables canned without added salt or sugar	Vegetables canned with salt and/or sugar
	Plain frozen vegetables	Frozen vegetables in sauces
	Fresh potatoes	Frozen french fries, potatoes in batter
Drinks	Fruit juices (fresh and reconstituted)	Fruit-flavored drinks
	Naturally carbonated fruit juices and mineral water with added juice	Sodas with added sugar or artificial sweeteners, colors, and flavors
Dairy produce	Mature and farmhouse cheeses	Processed cheeses and cheese slices
	Reduced-fat hard cheeses	Blue cheeses and some flavored cheeses
	Unsweetened low-fat or nonfat yogurt	Yogurt
	Real fruit yogurt	Fruit-flavored yogurt
	Skim and low-fat milk	Whole milk and milk with extra fat
	Dried skim milk	Dried milk with added fats

INDEX

ACKNOWLEDGMENTS

The publisher would like to thank the following
individuals and organizations for their
contribution to this book:

PHOTOGRAPHY

All photography by Peter Chadwick,
Andy Crawford, Andreas von Einsiedel, Steve
Gorton, Ranald Mackechnie, Jane Stockman,
Clive Streeter

NUTRITIONAL ADVICE

Jasmine Challis BSc, SRD

ADDITIONAL EDITORIAL ASSISTANCE

Nicky Adamson, Dawn Bates, Claire Cross,
David Summers

DTP ASSISTANCE

Rajen Shah

INDEX

Hilary Bird

TEXT FILM

The Brightside Partnership, London